Cheng Man-ch'ing and T'ai Chi

Echoes in the Hall of Happiness

An
Anthology
of Articles
from the
*Journal of
Asian Martial Arts*

Edited by Michael A. DeMarco, M.A.
& T. G. LaFredo, MFA

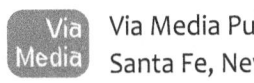

Via Media Publishing
Santa Fe, New Mexico

Disclaimer
Please note that the authors and publisher of this book are not responsible in any manner whatsoever for any injury that may result from practicing the techniques and/or following the instructions given within. Since the physical activities described herein may be too strenuous in nature for some readers to engage in safely, it is essential that a physician be consulted prior to training.

All Rights Reserved
No part of this publication, including illustrations, may be reproduced or utilized in any form or by any means, electronic or mechanical, including photocopying, recording, or by any information storage and retrieval system (beyond that copying permitted by sections 107 and 108 of the US Copyright Law and except by reviewers for the public press), without written permission from Via Media Publishing Company.

Warning: Any unauthorized act in relation to a copyright work may result in both a civil claim for damages and criminal prosecution.

Copyright © 2015 by
Via Media Publishing Company
941 Calle Mejia #822
Santa Fe, NM 87501 USA
E-mail: md@goviamedia.com

All articles in this anthology were originally published
in the *Journal of Asian Martial Arts*.
Listed according to the table of contents for this anthology:

Davis, B. (1996)	Volume 5, Number 2	pages 36–59
Sutton, N. (1994)	Volume 3, Number 1	pages 56–71
Smith, R. (1995)	Volume 4, Number 1	pages 50–65
Smith, R. (1995)	Volume 4, Number 1	pages 46–59
Smith, R. (1997)	Volume 6, Number 1	pages 50–61
Smith, R. (1997)	Volume 6, Number 2	pages 56–69
Mason, R. et al. (2010)	Volume 19, Number 2	pages 72–107
Davis, D. & Mann, L. (1996)	Volume 5, Number 4	pages 46–67
Mason, R. (2008)	Volume 17, Number 3	pages 22–39

Book and cover design by Via Media Publishing Company
Edited by Michael A. DeMarco, M.A., and T. G. LaFredo, MFA
Cover illustration: Michael Lane (www.golfandsportsbylane.com)

Cheng Man-ch'ing and T'ai Chi: Echoes in the Hall of Happiness/An Anthology
1. Martial arts–History. 2. Martial arts–Social and cultural aspects.
I. Title. II. Cheng Man-ch'ing/Zheng Manqing

ISBN-13: 978-1-893765-06-1 (alk. paper)

www.viamediapublishing.com

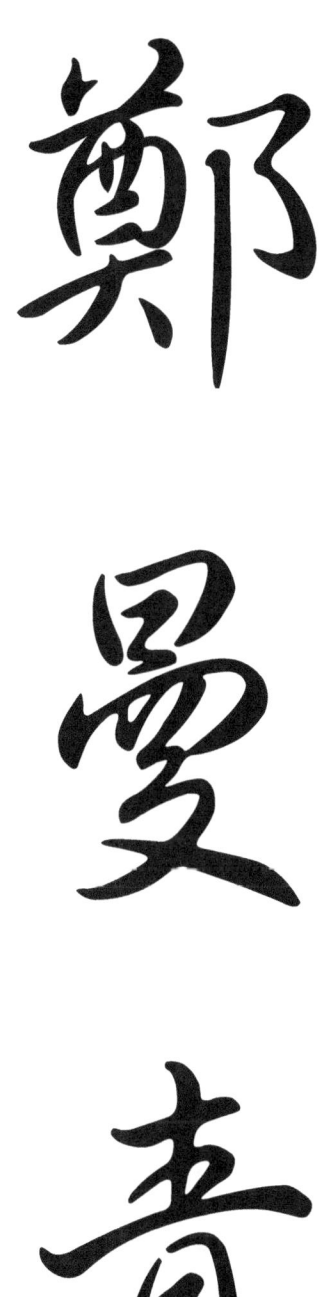

contents

v **Preface**
Michael DeMarco, M.A.

viii **Author Bio Notes**

CHAPTERS

1 In Search of a Unified Dao:
Zheng Manqing's Life and Contribution to Taijiquan
Barbara Davis, M.A.

31 The Development of Zheng Manqing Taijiquan in Malaysia
Nigel Sutton, M.A.

49 Zheng Manqing and Taijiquan: A Clarification of Role
Robert W. Smith, M.A.

68 Remembering Zheng Manqing: Some Sketches from His Life
Robert W. Smith, M.A.

86 Chen Weiming, Zheng Manqing, and the Difference between Strength and Intrinsic Energy
Robert W. Smith, M.A.

101 Dalü and Some Tigers
Robert W. Smith, M.A.

113 Liu Xiheng: Memories of a Taiji Sage
Contributions by Benjamin Lo, Xu Yizhong, Yuan Weiming, Xu Zhengmei, & Danny Emerick. Compiled by Russ Mason, M.A.

148 Conservator of the *Taiji Classics*:
An Interview with Benjamin Pangjeng Lo
Donald D. Davis, Ph.D. & Lawrence L. Mann

170 Zheng Manqing: The Memorial Hall and Legacy of the Master of Five Excellences in Taiwan
Russ Mason, M.A.

196 **Index**

preface

Note: There are many systems used to transliterate Chinese to the Latin alphabet, but the academic standard and official phonetic system in China used today is known as Pinyin. All should be using this method, but we have a few hundred years of familiarity with older systems that persist in common usage today. We have decided to keep the more familiar "Cheng Man-ch'ing" and "t'ai chi" spellings for this book's title because they are widely recognized. For the main text, however, Chinese names and terms are in Pinyin.

Zheng Manqing (1902–1975)—also known by the more familiar romanization Cheng Man-ch'ing—certainly played a lead role in popularizing taijiquan throughout the world and greatly influencing the way the art is perceived and practiced. This fact alone should drive all those interested in taiji to study the man's history and thought.

There is a huge body of writings and video representations of Zheng's taiji theory and practice. Unfortunately, much of the available content actually obscures Zheng's message. The result is that Zheng and his role in taiji evolution are often not fully understood and faulty conclusions are made. A further result is that many feel either enlightened with what they believe to be true, or they become even more perplexed in who Zheng was as a human and what his taiji truly embodied.

The chapters in this anthology contain rare information about Professor Zheng not available elsewhere, except in their originally published formats in the *Journal of Asian Martial Arts*. Most of the articles in the journal were written in an academic style, limiting their acceptance from the general public, which is typically interested in the more accessible popular writing styles. Of course the content here deals not only with the complexities of taiji theory and practice, but does so in a thick weave of historical and cultural threads.

We are republishing the journal articles in book format so all with a sincere interest in taiji history, theory, and practice can benefit from the content, particularly those interested in the Zheng Manqing tradition. Each author is uniquely qualified for producing some of the highest-quality writings in this specialized area.

Articles are not presented in chronological order according to their original publication dates, but are assembled to give a detailed look at the life and teachings of Professor Zheng. Barbara Davis's work appears first because it gives a thorough overview of Zheng's life and thought, plus the significance of the historical and cultural milieu that nurtured this Renaissance man.

Zheng Manqing lived in mainland China, Taiwan, and the US. He conducted most of his taiji teaching in Taiwan and the US, so many are familiar with him in these areas. Zheng did travel to Malaysia. His influence is strong there because one of his senior students, Huang Xingxian, moved to Singapore, then to Malaysia from Taiwan. Thanks to Nigel Sutton, chapter 2 provides a perspective on Zheng's influence in Malaysia. His viewpoints may differ from the perspectives of those closely connected to Zheng through the US lineage. For this reason, you should find his comments thoughtfully stimulating. His experience and analysis help to jar some of the common beliefs associated with Zheng's teaching and practice. He gives us reason to pause and question what can really be known about Zheng and the development of his art as it dispersed around the world.

The next four articles are all by Robert W. Smith, who many believe was the leading authority on Zheng Manqing and his taiji. His first article, "A Clarification of Role," was written in response to Sutton's article. There is no smooth yin-yang harmony here, but a healthy polemic for refining our views of Zheng and the theory and practice of taijiquan.

The following three chapters by Smith add some details of Professor Zheng's life and his particular flavor of taiji. His discussions on energy, push-hands, and *dalü*, should benefit all readers by his insights and speculation. These chapters are followed by works that highlight the lives and teachings of two of Zheng's most senior representatives: Liu Xiheng and Benjamin Pangjeng Lo.

Russ Mason compiled a fine tribute to Liu Xiheng. In addition to his own contribution to this work, he enriched the piece with wonderful reflections by Ben Lo, Xu Yizhong, Yuan Weiming, Xu Zhengmei, and Danny Emerick. The result is the most thorough presentation in English dealing with Zheng's protégé, who headed his school in Taiwan after Zheng moved to the US. Known for his exquisite touch in push-hands and swordplay, Liu was likewise admired for his refined character.

We are fortunate to have another piece that, like the thoroughness found in Mason's chapter, offers a highly insightful interview with Benjamin Lo. Lo was Professor Zheng's first student in Taiwan. He is a primary representative of Zheng's taiji, having spread the practice in the US since immigrating in 1974. His publications and teachings on the *Taiji Classics* have benefited practitioners around the world. The interview by Davis and Mann draws out Lo's thoughts on taiji theory and practice, and his memories of Professor Zheng. His advice for taiji players—tempered by his decades of practice as demanded by old-school tradition—provides rare insights for modern practitioners.

This anthology is capped off with an appropriate piece by Russ Mason, following his visit to the Zheng Manqing Memorial Hall in Taiwan. He recounts the accomplishments of the Master of Five Excellences (traditional Chinese medicine, martial arts, and the fine arts of painting, poetry, and calligraphy). In addition to highlighting major aspects of the Professor's life, Mason escorts us through Zheng's former residence turned memorial hall, where we see the desk where Zheng worked, displays of paintings and poetry, and personal items from his daily life. This chapter brings a sense of the man's presence—a true memorial hall.

We are thrilled to publish this anthology, knowing it provides some of the best materials available about Zheng Manqing and his taiji. Much credit goes to each of the authors for their years of research and for their time devoted to capturing valued content so others can benefit from the reading. The main body of text forming each chapter is supported by notes, bibliographies, and illustrations that are likewise valuable and conveniently assembled in one book.

The Master of Five Excellences departed the earthly realm on March 26, 1975. For all interested in taiji, Zheng's genius should not be forgotten, but regularly referred to for insight and inspiration today. In the same vein, we offer this anthology assembled from selected articles from the *Journal of Asian Martial Arts*—a trove of specialized works dealing with all aspects of the Asian martial traditions. The chapters here include all the content as presented in the journal articles, so you may notice a few duplicate illustrations. We hope this first anthology will stimulate further research into the Zheng Manqing tradition, and steer practitioners toward many years of health-nurturing taiji practice.

Michael A. DeMarco
Santa Fe
August 2015

author bio notes

Barbara Davis, M.A., has a master's degree in East Asian studies from the University of Minnesota. She trained in Taiwan and the United States with senior students of the late Professor Zheng Manqing, including Maggie Newman, Ed Young, Liu Xiheng of Taibei, and in workshops with Ben Lo. She produced the quarterly *Taijiquan Journal* for nearly five years, and is the author of *The Taijiquan Classics: An Annotated Translation* (Blue Snake Books, 2004), and translator of *Taiji Sword* by Chen Weiming (Blue Snake Books, 2000).

Donald Davis, Ph.D., earned a doctorate in psychology from Michigan State University. He has also served as a faculty member in the Institute of Asian Studies at Old Dominion University in Norfolk, Virginia. Dr. Davis teaches taiji and Daoism at Tidewater Tai Chi Center, carrying on the teachings of Robert W. Smith and Ben Lo.

Michael DeMarco, M.A., received his degree from Seton Hall University's Asian Studies Department. In 1964 he began studies of Indonesian kuntao-silat. Since 1973 he has focused on taijiquan: Yang style, Xiong Yanghe lineage; Chen style, Du Yuze lineage. He founded Via Media Publishing Company in 1991, producing the *Journal of Asian Martial Arts* and books. He teaches taiji in Santa Fe, New Mexico.

T. G. LaFredo, MFA, earned his master's degree in creative writing from Antioch University Los Angeles. He served as copyeditor of the *Journal of Asian Martial Arts* from December 2009 through the final issue and continues with Via Media Publishing's other endeavors.

Lawrence L. Mann (d. 1997) founded the Tidewater Tai Chi Center in 1974 in Virginia Beach, Virginia, where he carried on the teachings of Robert W. Smith and Ben Lo.

Russ Mason, M.A., TESL, received his degree from Oklahoma State University, teaches language and culture at the University of Delaware, and has taught taijiquan for the University of Delaware's College of Health and Nursing Science and Confucius Institute. He began training in Yang-style taijiquan in the 1970s in the lineage of Professor Zheng Manqing, initially with Dr. B. A. Fusaro. His primary teachers were Robert W. Smith (US) and Liu Xiheng (Taiwan).

Robert W. Smith, M.A., received a master's degree from the University of Washington in Seattle. He was a pioneer in Asian martial arts research in America with fourteen published books and numerous articles. From his late teens he trained under eminent Western boxing and wrestling coaches and later immersed himself in judo and finally taiji under Zheng Manqing. He taught many students in the Washington, DC, area, where he worked as an intelligence officer for the CIA. Smith shared more than fifty years' experience in martial arts practice and research in *Martial Musings: A Portrayal of Martial Arts in the Twentieth Century* (Via Media Publishing, 1999).

Nigel Sutton, M.A., has studied martial arts since he was thirteen years old and has trained extensively and intensively with a number of different teachers in the Zheng Manqing branch of taijiquan in Malaysia, plus others in the arts of silat, Chen taiji, and eskrima. He currently lives in Malaysia, where he makes a living as a writer. This is also the location for the Zhong Ding Training Academy in Penang, where Nigel delivers residential training courses. His book titles include *Tai Chi Roots & Branches* (Tuttle, 1996) and *Applied Tai Chi Chuan* (Tuttle, 1998).

In Search of a Unified Dao: Zheng Manqing's Life and Contribution to Taijiquan
by Barbara Davis, M.A.

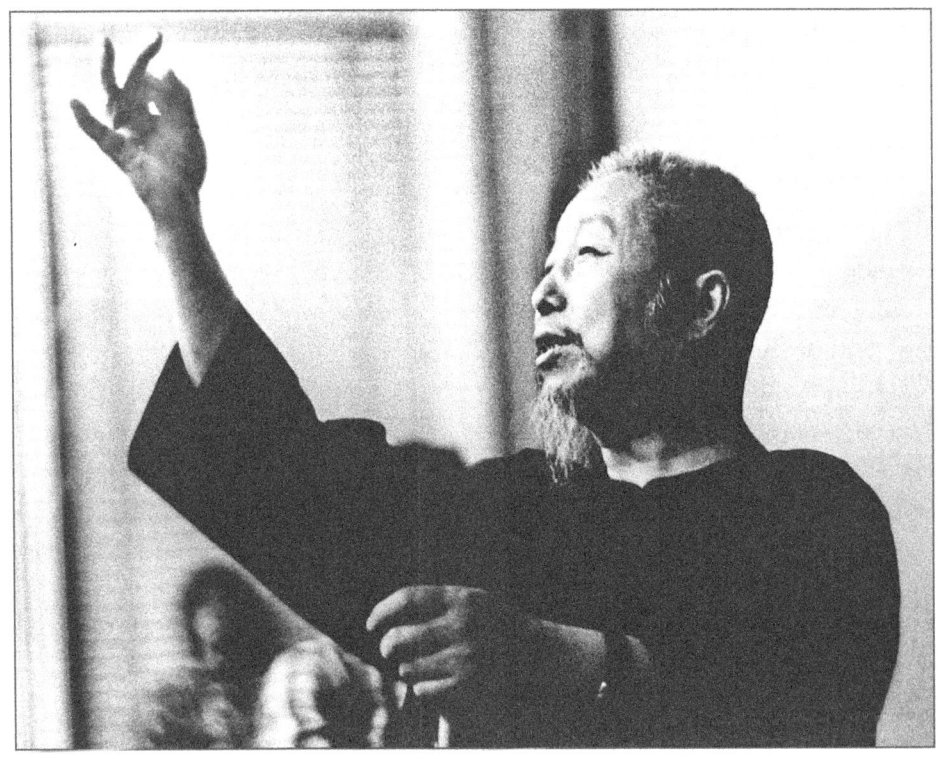

Zheng Manqing lecturing at the Shizhong (a.k.a. Shr Jung) school in New York City, where he delivered a number of talks on taijiquan, philosophy, and health.
All photos courtesy of Ken van Sickle, except where noted.

In little over 150 years, taijiquan has grown from being a family-held tradition in a small village in northern China to become an international phenomenon. Of the many people who have been involved with its growth in the twentieth century and in its movement to the West, one of the most influential figures was Zheng Manqing.

Like his predecessors in the Yang family lineage, Zheng was instrumental in helping taijiquan reach new audiences. His erudition, skill, personality, and his social connections all helped in this. Zheng brought to his teachings a thorough knowledge of several disciplines, and to his writing a depth of classical learning that the taijiquan world had until then not seen.

As a result, Zheng Manqing indisputably has had a great impact on how many of us now think about and practice taijiquan. Now, decades after Zheng Manqing's death, it is helpful for us to examine the details of his life and the cultural and historical environment that nurtured his ideas, so we may better understand his unique contributions to the world of taijiquan. As many readers may not be familiar with the full scope of his writings, an extensive bibliography has been appended that lists Zheng's many works, and those written about him.

The World of Traditional China

To talk about Zheng Manqing, or any Chinese traditionalist for that matter, we must start with Confucius. Over 2,400 years ago, the great sage said to his disciples, "My Dao is that of an all-pervading unity." These deceptively simple words (yet so difficult to implement) became a motto for his followers throughout the centuries, including the young Zheng Manqing.

Confucius's ideas are rooted in humanism, and are expressed in proper behavior and relationships. After his time, his ideas became codified in traditions, curricula, and laws. He is revered in China as "the First Teacher." He promoted respect for the ancients, broad learning, and careful reflection. Confucius and his teachings became the very symbol of traditional China, and had a profound impact on all aspects of Chinese society and that of much of East Asia.

A twentieth-century paragon of Confucius's teachings, Zheng also became a teacher, one who welcomed all who were serious about study, regardless of nationality. He emphasized in all of his work an unrelenting quest for the ideals of Confucius and his early interpreter, Mencius.

However, by the time Zheng was born, at the beginning of the twentieth century, the traditional society that Confucian ideas had so influenced was crumbling away, torn from inside and outside by the forces of change and modernization. Yet throughout his life, Zheng remained drawn to the world of the traditional scholar, or literati, a world steeped in poetry, art, philosophy, and history.

Zheng and his peers struggled to understand their circumstance at the turbulent nexus of tradition and modernity. Many chose to cast away the old ways and pursue Western-influenced sciences and social structures in hopes of building a new society that would be unfettered by the weight of history and tradition. On the other extreme, for many traditionally minded people, the task was one of accepting the dominant trends toward modernization, but maintaining and utilizing the strengths of the past. Zheng argued for this latter ideal his whole life.

Zheng wove together his many talents and interests with seeming ease, untiringly guiding others. He followed the Dao, or Way, of Confucianism, which emphasized above all else human relations. Zheng coupled this with an unswerving loyalty to family, friends, students, and country.

Accomplished at painting, poetry, calligraphy, taijiquan, and medicine, Zheng was known in his later years by the sobriquet Master of Five Excellences. Today his followers still respectfully refer to him as "the Professor," and he is recognized around the world for his contributions to taijiquan. In Taiwan in particular, his paintings and calligraphy are prized possessions. Among his students, friends, and patients, his medical skills were considered superb and subtle. Beyond these accomplishments, he is remembered by many as an eloquent and gifted teacher and writer. His wide-ranging interests and multiple talents provided him with a rich ground for cross-fertilization of ideas. These talents, together with the circumstances of his life, presented him with opportunities to make unique and influential contributions.

Even now, decades after his death in 1975, Zheng Manqing has continued to accumulate taijiquan followers through his books and through the continued efforts of his direct and indirect students. But what made Zheng so influential? What was unique about his work? To answer these questions, we will first look at the life and surroundings of this multidimensional man.

Zheng Manqing's Life

Zheng was born in the waning years of the Qing dynasty, on July 29, 1902.[2] His given name was Yue. He later took the name Manqing (Man-ch'ing), and used Manran (Man-jan, "Beautiful Whiskers") in his fifties.[3] He often used pen names in concert with these names, including Hermit of the Jade Well, Host of the Tower of Long Evening, and Old One Who Never Tires of Learning.[4]

Zheng was a native of the Yongia district in the fertile province of Zhejiang (Chekiang), on the southeast coast of China. This small port town and surrounding district, all now known as Wenzhou, is on the mouth of the Ou River, a short distance from the coast of the East China Sea.[5]

Zheng was the youngest of six children.[6] His father died when he was very young, and the family was poor.[7] Zheng's mother's surname was Zhang.[8] During his childhood, she taught him herbal medicine, calligraphy, and poetry. He tells that when he was a child, he would tug at her sleeve and plead with her to recite Tang dynasty poetry to him.[9] When he was six, she began to teach him calligraphy. Her sister, Zhang Guang, also known as Old Lady Redfern, was a painter of some renown who later helped him develop his skills at the "outline" style of painting.[10]

Zheng was precocious and had a photographic memory, but his childhood was also marked by illnesses and a major accident. When he was nine, he was hit in the head with a brick from a crumbling wall and fell into a coma for several days. When he came to, he had lost his memory. To help him recuperate, the family used herbal remedies, and then apprenticed him to a local painter, Wang Xiangchan, in hope that simple work like grinding the painter's ink would be therapeutic.[11] As he recuperated, the many hours in the studio made a lasting impression on the young boy, and he began to practice painting, at first on leftover paper wrappers from his grandmother's medicines.

By the age of fourteen, Zheng had mastered painting well enough that his teacher sent him out on his own. In the traditional manner, Wang gave him a studio name (Wisteria Flower) and set prices for his paintings, thereby initiating him into a professional life that would span decades and continents. Zheng spent the next several years in nearby Hangzhou, a renowned center of the arts, where he studied painting, poetry, and calligraphy. He was soon able to support his family by means of his artwork. Even in these early years, his painting favored the expressive *xieyi* style of brushwork; as for subjects, he concentrated primarily on flowers and plants.[12]

When he was seventeen, Zheng went to Beijing. It was 1919, just as the May Fourth reform movement was reaching its height. This movement was made up of students and intellectuals who questioned the old structures of governance, education, and society. They sought to open up China to new ideas from Japan, Europe, and the United States, in an effort to shed what they thought of as a stagnant past. They also promoted the use of vernacular Chinese in writing, rather than the classical Chinese that had been the mainstay of the written word since long before Confucius.

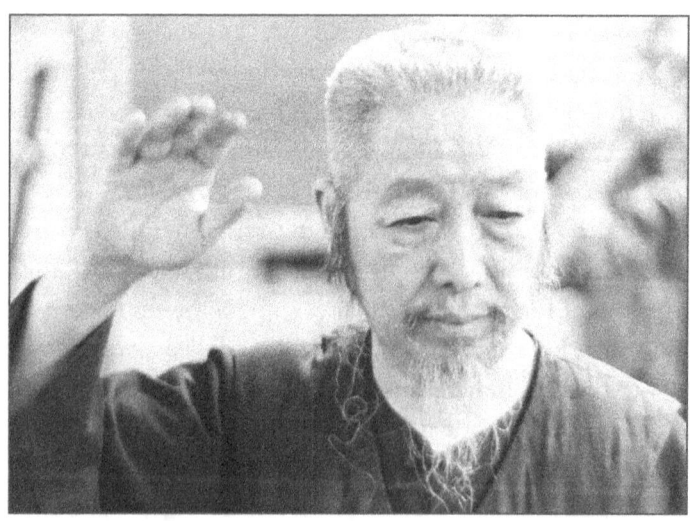

Zheng Manqing moving through the taiji forms.

In Beijing, Zheng became a member of several circles of poets and painters, who were for the most part older gentlemen of a traditionalist bent. These connections eventually led to an invitation to teach poetry at Yuwen University in 1924. That same year, Cai Yuanpei, chancellor of Beijing University and a fellow native of Zhejiang Province, recommended him for a teaching position at National Zhinan University in Shanghai.[13] In Shanghai, Zheng was invited to be director of the painting department at the Shanghai School of Fine Arts and was later involved with the start up of the College of Culture and Art. In 1925 he had a solo art show at the Shuixie Pavilion in Beijing's Central Park, and was sent by the Ministry of Education to Japan to do research on the arts. The next year, he assembled his first collection of paintings.[14]

Zheng began to study medicine more rigorously in his midtwenties. Building on the base that he had gained from his mother, he began to study around 1926 with Dr. Song You'an of Anhui Province, whom he had met in Shanghai. His medical training encompassed both practice and theory, and became a major part of his livelihood, as well as an important aspect of his understanding of taijiquan.

Zheng had a weakened body since childhood. He contracted tuberculosis while in Beijing, and still was suffering from it when he went to live in Shanghai. When a friend suggested he take up taijiquan to regain his health, Zheng assented. Earlier in his life he had studied some taijiquan as well as exercises such as *baduanjin* and *yijinjing* in efforts to strengthen himself.[15]

In the mid-1920s, Yang Chengfu (1883–1936), one of the well-known members of the Yang family lineage of taijiquan, began teaching in Shanghai with his senior disciple Chen Weiming (1881–1958). They founded the Zhi Rou [Attaining Softness] Taijiquan Society.[16] In 1932 Zheng Manqing was introduced by an acquaintance to Yang Chengfu and commenced close to six years of study with Yang.[17] Zheng won Master Yang's favor after healing Yang's wife from a serious illness. At her urging, Yang taught Zheng without holding anything back. Zheng was a quick learner, and after only a year made great progress. Zheng also briefly studied with Zhang Qinlin, who was from Taiyuan, Shanxi Province.[18]

By 1930 Professor Zheng had retired from college teaching, and spent time in neighboring Jiangsu Province, where he studied essay and poem writing with Qian Mingshan.[19] He was soon able to put his improved writing skills to good use, as Yang Chengfu called upon him to write a preface for, and, as many assert, to ghostwrite Yang's 1934 book *Taijiquan tiyong quan shu*.[20] Zheng's preface draws in ideas from the *Yijing*, the *Book of Songs*, and the *Daodejing* among others, demonstrating his early efforts to synthesize classical learning with taijiquan. In his hands, taijiquan was not merely exercise or boxing. It was part of the Confucian Dao he so admired.

The War Years

In 1895 the Japanese took control of southern Manchuria and Taiwan, and forced many humiliating concessions from the Chinese. The encroachments continued until 1937, when the Japanese launched a brutal war against the Chinese. This lasted until the Japanese surrender at the end of World War II. The two main players in China, the Communists and the Nationalists (the Kuomintang or Guomindang), were able to put aside their differences for a time to unite against their common enemy. But as soon as peace was declared on the international front, full-scale civil war broke out at home. At the time the Sino-Japanese War began, Zheng Manqing was practicing medicine full time. He had previously taught taijiquan at the Central Military Academy (formerly named Huangpu or Whampoa) in 1933. He now assisted the military in the war efforts by teaching taijiquan in Hunan (for the provincial government) and Sichuan (for the Central Military Training Group), and by writing medical prescriptions useful to the military.

The Nationalist government relocated westward to Chongqing in 1939, in Sichuan Province. Zheng moved along with it. Now thirty-seven, he continued to practice traditional medicine and teach taijiquan. With his colleagues he formed and then served as president of the National Chinese Medical Association. This group's purpose was to help promote traditional medicine, which was under attack by modernizers enamored of Western science and medicine. Zheng served as a member of the National Assembly for the Construction of the Constitution in 1946, and as a representative for the Community of Doctors of Traditional Medicine to the National Assembly in 1947. He married Ding Yidu when he was forty. She was the daughter of an Air Force official and had studied medicine at Beijing University. Together they had five children: three girls and two boys.

It was during this period that Zheng worked on condensing the hundred-some moves of the Yang family taijiquan form he had learned from Yang Chengfu down to thirty-seven moves. In 1946, while still in Nanjing, he completed work on his first taijiquan book, *Zhengzi taijiquan shisan pian* [Master Zheng's Thirteen Treatises on Taijiquan]. This book was aimed at the serious practitioner and in its first part delved into the deeper philosophy and medical substantiations for taijiquan practice. The second part was a thorough examination of the martial application of the moves, along with photographs. The war interfered, however, and the manuscript was not published until 1950, when Zheng and his family were safely in Taiwan. The book received support from high places. Among its calligraphed dedications are ones by President Chiang Kai-shek, Control Yuan President Yu Youren, and elder classmate Chen Weiming. Chen's support was particularly important, due to his high status among Yang Chengfu's senior students and as a well-educated early taijiquan writer himself.[21]

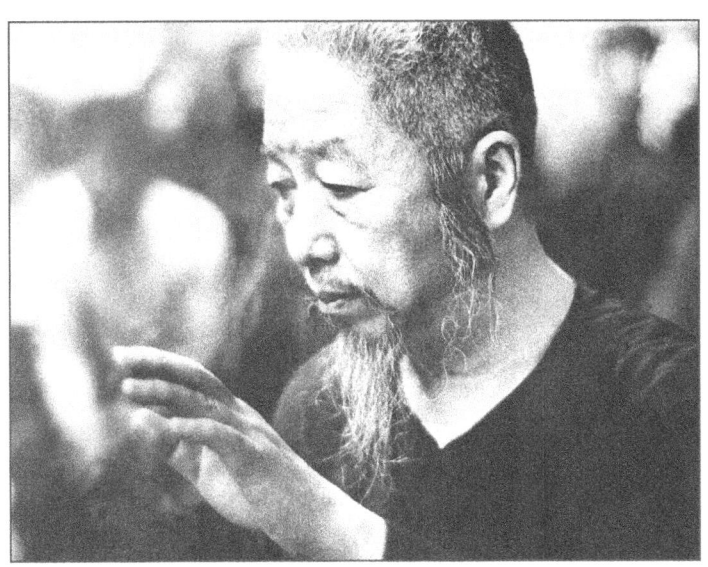

Zheng Manqing moving through the taiji forms.

In Taiwan

The Nationalist government was to relocate yet one more time. When the mainland fell to the Communists, millions of people who had been connected to the Nationalist effort took refuge on the island province of Taiwan, a hundred miles off the southeast coast of China. The nationalist governmental seat was now activated in Taibei. Under the guidance of Chiang Kai-shek and the Guomindang, a governing body for all of China—in absentia—was put in place. The civil war ostensibly over, a cold war ensued, with martial law kept in place on the island until 1987.

The mainland refugees considered Taiwan to be a temporary haven until the mainland was retaken. From behind the cold war barricade, the Nationalist refugees turned toward developing Taiwan economically, creating a free China that would prove their politics correct. The Nationalist government presented itself in international politics as the "true China," holding the much-coveted United Nations seat until 1971. They continued to seek and receive United States aid, and served as an important outpost and staging ground for it in the Korean and Vietnam conflicts.

In this atmosphere of resettlement, Zheng Manqing quickly reestablished a sense of normalcy. He started new poetry and calligraphy circles, and became involved with the national arts scene by helping to start and run the Republic of China Fine Arts Society. One of his more influential painting students was Madame Chiang Kai-shek. He was invited to teach poetry, painting, and calligraphy at the graduate school of the College of Chinese Culture in Taibei.

Zheng taught taijiquan publicly for several years at the request of the Taibei mayor. Usually, however, students came to him via personal introductions. If they did not yet know the taijiquan form, a more senior student would be assigned to teach it to them. Students would gather informally on the weekends to work out in the courtyard of his home in Yonghe (a Taibei suburb). Zheng titled his group the Shizhong [Correct Timing] Taijiquan Center, which continues to operate to this day under the guidance of his direct students.

In 1961, at the age of sixty, Zheng published his second collection of paintings, *Manran xieyi*, as well as a short work on gynecology and his first volume of poetry. In 1962, perhaps sensing the future of taijiquan's growth, he published an English instructional book, *Taijiquan for Health and Self-Defense*, through the Shizhong Center. This book, aimed at the beginner, illustrated his simplified form and articulated his philosophy of taijiquan. In 1965 a Chinese book, *Zhengzi taijiquan zixiu xinfa* [Master Zheng's New Method of Taijiquan Self-Cultivation] came out. This book described the moves in detail, with photographs and foot charts, and also contained a reprint of the thirteen chapters previously published in *Zheng Zi taijiquan shisan pian* [Master Zheng's Thirteen Treatises on Taijiquan]. In 1967 he published a second English-language text, *T'ai Chi*, in collaboration with his student Robert W. Smith, an American martial arts historian.

Like many of his contemporaries in Taiwan, Zheng felt the pain of separation from his family. Torn from each other by years of war and exile, his writing showed little of his feelings. It is only in his poetry that the depth of this hurt and the conflicts it raised are revealed, as is shown in "Receiving a Letter from Home":

> After New Year's a letter from home arrives
> My soul is cut off from a dream, it is difficult to return.
> My younger brother has died from who knows what illness,
> Mother is aging, with no one to lean on,
> In her desolate hut, tries to make a living from a tiny piece of land,
> Passing the days, suffering unending hunger.
> In the waning night, in tears longing for her son,
> Sobbing, not daring to wipe away the tears.[23]

A low-grade state of war was still in effect between the mainland People's Republic of China and the Taiwan-based Republic of China. There was no way for him or others to communicate directly with their families left behind on the mainland. This sense of isolation and loss, combined with the terrible weight of not being able to fulfill their filial duties toward their parents, was a burden never resolved for many of his generation who found themselves in exile.

The American Years

In 1964 Zheng travelled to Europe and the United States to mount exhibits of his artwork. He had a one-man show in Paris at the Cernuschi Museum of Chinese Art, and then exhibited at the Republic of China pavilion at the New York World's Fair. While in the United States he gave a demonstration of taijiquan at the United Nations, and met up with many old friends from the Chinese mainland. One of these friends encouraged him to stay in New York City so as to be able to write and teach.[24] Zheng decided to settle in Manhattan with his family and yet again he set about establishing venues for his practice of medicine, painting, and taijiquan. Within a short time of his arrival in New York City, he had established the Shizhong Center for Culture and the Arts in Chinatown with the help of local sponsors. This center soon became the locus of many of his activities. It was here that he taught taijiquan, saw patients, and gave lectures.

Zheng was one of taijiquan's earliest and foremost proponents overseas. He said, "I not only desire my country to be strong, I would also like to share the benefits of taijiquan with all mankind."[25] He willingly taught non-Chinese as well as his fellow countrymen, men and women equally, and made full use of his books, lectures, articles, and even movies to disseminate his ideas.

The Shizhong Center, initially on Canal Street in Chinatown, quickly began to attract an interesting mix of students.[26] Word had passed quickly around in both Chinese and martial arts circles that a taijiquan master had come to town. Among his early students were overseas Chinese, who ranged from businessmen to restaurant workers. There were many Americans, including serious martial artists, as well as a large number of hippies.

Zheng seemed to care deeply for his students, regardless of their nationality, and treated their foibles with a sense of amusement. He seized the chance to influence them, both in the Chinese tradition of teacher as surrogate parent, and as a representative of Chinese culture.

Now in his sixties, Zheng had come to the United States at a time when many American youth were rebelling against their parents and teachers, and against the draft and the war in Vietnam. Demonstrations and fierce political debates were commonplace, as were "free love" and the use of drugs. Anyone in a position of authority—or anyone over thirty—was automatically suspect.

Into this social turmoil walked Zheng, who, as a "master from the Far East," could neatly sidestep this politicized atmosphere. His physical appearance—a slight sixty-five-year-old man in Chinese scholar's robes with a graying crew cut and sparse, long whiskers—did not fit the young Americans' image of one of their own authoritarian elders. Besides, he was different: he was an artist, poet, and herbalist.

Ironically, the traditions these American students were so eager to absorb from Zheng were at the same time being violently rejected by their counterparts in China. Mao Zedong's Cultural Revolution in the People's Republic of China was underway, and its destructiveness was not known yet in the West. Zheng also avoided the controversy over American involvement in Vietnam. Though many of his American students were involved in leftist antiwar protests, and he himself was an ardent anticommunist, Zheng steered clear of public debate.

Toward his Chinese students and friends, Zheng's mission was slightly different. He viewed it as his responsibility to help keep traditional culture alive for them, and to keep them engaged with it. He frequently wrote of the importance of keeping Chinese youth linked to their moral and ethical roots.[27]

In Zheng's hands, taijiquan and the Shizhong Center became vehicles for the promotion of Chinese culture.[28] With the help of translators, he taught taijiquan and delivered lectures on Confucius's *Doctrine of the Mean*, Laozi's *Daodejing*, and health. Beyond taijiquan study, philosophy, art, and culture, students also unconsciously absorbed Chinese attitudes about the teacher-student and student-student hierarchy. These relationships to some extent replicate Chinese family structure, with the teacher as parent. For example, when teaching in New York City, Zheng did not hesitate to comment on the length of the male American students' hair, and when one of the more serious students cut his hair, Zheng observed that he had become more human.[29]

Many of Zheng's students revered him. Zheng advised them on their marriages, jobs, and health. They would come, as did many nonstudents, to consult with him on health matters. He would sit at his desk at the studio, read their pulses, and then write out a prescription for them to have filled at the nearby Chinese herbal pharmacies.

Zheng knew of the temptations of the free love and drugs with which the students were surrounded. He knew how poor the American diet and lifestyle was, and taught them about the need for balance of food and rest. He recognized their search for answers to the upheaval in society and their own lives. He talked to them about the Dao, giving them answers to questions that at the time they themselves didn't even realize they were asking.

Zheng painted at his study in his home, which was high up in an apartment building on Riverside Drive in the Upper West Side. He named his study Tower of the Long Twilight for its view of the sunset over the Hudson River. The curator of his Parisian exhibit praised his work, saying Zheng Manqing, "more than any of his contemporaries, pushed to its extreme limits the role played by the discipline of the mind. His entire work is suffused by the unmistakable strength of his brush."[30] In 1967 Zheng wrote on one of his paintings of bamboo with what had by then become his characteristic blunt-tipped calligraphic style:

> Painting is like catching a fleeting glimpse of a galloping
> white horse through a crack. In communicating one's spirit,
> the brush must move as if chasing the wind.[31]

Zheng Manqing held to traditional culture through all of his years away from China. Even after close to ten years of living in New York City, he still maintained his traditional scholar's appearance. He had a sense of the importance of tradition and held to Confucius's admiration of the past, as shown in this poem from 1973:

> Whose brush can excel both old and new?
> With every rub of my eyes I recognize the distant hills anew.
> Last night a clear dream inspired a poetic thought.
> The single stroke of the green mountain
> Contains all my heart's yearning for antiquity.[32]

At the same time, Zheng noted in his painting essays that there were those artists who felt that an overadmiration of the ancients (in this case, painters) stifled innovation and ignored today's masters. To admire past masters did not mean to be "mired in traditionalism." Rather, one should build on a solid foundation of understanding the past, and that ultimately, it was most important to follow Nature.[33]

Zheng received the title of director of fine arts, the Republic of China Cultural Renaissance Movement, American Branch. The Renaissance Movement, initiated by Chiang Kai-shek, aimed to reinforce traditional culture and all its values, as a response to the destructive forces of Mao Zedong's Cultural Revolution. The Nationalists felt themselves to be protectors and guardians of traditional Chinese culture and its treasures, and later felt a sense of vindication when the true devastation of the Cultural Revolution became known.[34]

Even under criticism from some of his friends, Zheng continued to write in classical Chinese his whole life.[35] Language had been a part of the cultural battleground in China from the early 1900s. Educational and governmental reforms brought to an end the monopoly that classical Chinese had over the written language, and ushered in a flowering of vernacular writing. But for some traditionalists such as Zheng, the written language was sacrosanct, and to become cut off linguistically from the wellsprings of the past was a grave mistake.

Zheng wrote copiously while in New York City. It was a time for reflection and distillation of his ideas, resulting in commentaries on the *Daodejing*; the

Confucian classics of the *Analects*, *Great Learning*, and *Doctrine of the Mean*; and the *Yijing*. A collection of his original essays on the arts, *Manran san lun* [Manran's three treatises], was published in 1974 in Taibei.[36] As one of his last books, *Manran san lun* brought together under one cover essays on three of his "excellences": painting, calligraphy, and poetry. Perhaps nowhere else is his ability to weave together his interests as visible as in this book. In his preface he remarks:

> Calligraphy and painting are rooted in the same source. [As is said of the early poet and painter] Wang Wei, "In his poems are paintings, and in his paintings are poems." Guang Wen's Three Excellences [painting, poetry, and calligraphy] came forth from the same hand, and met together on the same page, united by sentiment.[37]

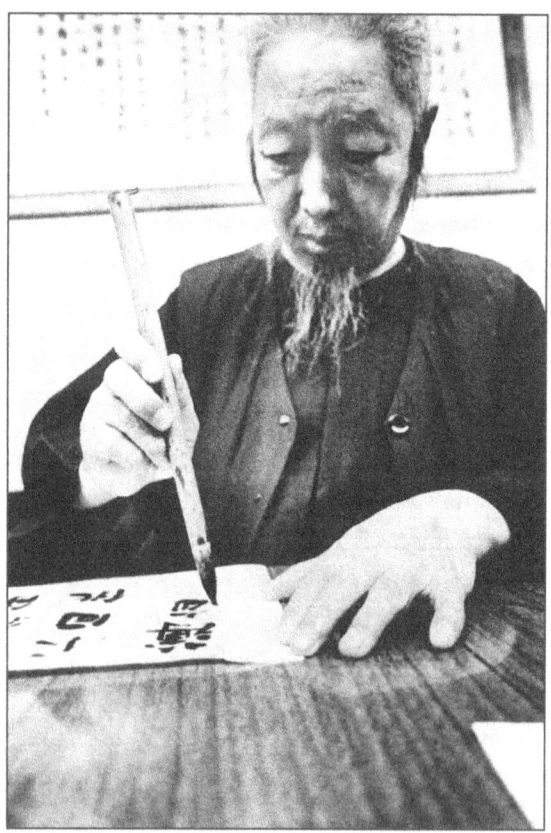

Zheng completing a poem. In China, well-developed calligraphic skills are highly respected. Calligraphy requires great inner concentration and control.

In the same preface, he links painting to the medical concepts so familiar to him as an herbal doctor:

> As for brush and ink, it is just like harmonizing the qi and blood. If the brush has too little ink, then it will be dry; if the ink has no brush [i.e., the ink is not used] it will congeal. In the same way that the qi is able to command the blood to move, we can see that the brush leads the ink's movement.[38]

In a similar fashion, Zheng's essays on calligraphy are permeated with taijiquan-like metaphors. In "Establishing the Foundation," he describes the formation of qi and strength using language that just as easily could be describing taijiquan:

> How does the calligrapher lay a foundation? Sink the qi to the *dantian*. The sole of the foot is planted in the ground, that's all. He moves his qi to his shoulder, elbow, wrist, the fingers, and then reaches the tip of the brush.[39]

Zheng himself never stopped studying. In fact, late in life he took the nickname the Old Man Who Never Tires of Learning. In his introduction to his *Yijing* commentary, Zheng said that in his search for the book's core ideas, he found the most primary one was *ren* or "human conduct." Zheng went on to lament that "to not see Confucius's Dao is like the sun and moon not shining, which is a misfortune for all of humankind."

Professor Zheng went back to Taiwan several times during his sojourn in the United States. On each trip he saw to the publication of his books, exhibited his artwork, and lectured on taijiquan, philosophy, and medicine. In 1974 Zheng planned to go for a third visit to Taiwan. He designated six senior students to run the New York Shizhong school in his absence.[41] Zheng left for Taiwan with his assistant Tam Gibbs to oversee publication of his commentary on the *Yijing* that had been the focus of his scholarly work for a number of years. After reading the proofs he paraphrased Confucius, that now, having finished the *Yijing*, he could die without regret.[42] Just ten days before his old acquaintance Chiang Kai-shek passed away, Zheng himself died of a cerebral hemorrhage, March 26, 1975.

Zheng Manqing's Legacy

Zheng was mourned by his family and many friends and students. At the funeral in Taibei, hundreds of mourners came and kowtowed at the memorial service. His family and representatives of the diverse groups of people with whom he had associated were all present: the highest circles of government and military, medical doctors, artists, and taijiquan colleagues and students. Floral wreaths and calligraphic banners mournfully sang praises of his "five excellences."[43] Students and friends also held memorial services in Singapore and New York.

In 1982 the National Palace Museum arranged with Zheng's widow for a retrospective exhibit, for which twenty-five of his paintings and works of calligraphy were selected. This was a great tribute to him, as the Palace Museum did not routinely exhibit modern artists. A catalogue of this exhibit was published for the occasion that included a reprint of a preface written by Madame Chiang Kai-shek to an earlier collection of his paintings.[44]

Since Zheng Manqing's death, his seminal works on taijiquan have been translated into other languages, and his students have carried on his mission of spreading taijiquan through their own work. Though it has been decades since Zheng passed away, his influence has continued to spread. Already there are thousands of third- and fourth-generation students practicing within his lineage, as well as thousands of adepts from other schools who rely on his writings for guidance in their taijiquan study. Zheng, along with other Nationalist colleagues, has also been "rehabilitated" in mainland China, so that one can now find him and his writings listed in martial arts materials.[45]

Zheng Manqing's Innovations in Taijiquan

The original role of martial arts study had been grueling professional training for men who would work as guards, bodyguards, or boxers. However, as the use of modern firearms grew, some martial arts began to shift from a primary focus on fighting application toward use for health and self-cultivation.

New methods of training evolved that did not require as high a level of time commitment, physical ability, or exertion. This was particularly true in the case of taijiquan, as its focus on softness and relaxation made it more appealing to a broader segment of the population, such as members of the educated elite and women. With this growth of interest, the martial arts became known as cultural treasures and as a means of defending national interests:

> Just as a segment of late Ming literati abandoned their traditional disdain for martial pursuits in the face of Manchu aggression, so a number of early twentieth century intellectuals embraced *guoshu* (Chinese martial arts) as part of a program of self-strengthening to counter Japanese imperialism and Western models of modernization.[46]

Taijiquan changed to fit into the social climate of the late Qing and early Republic, even in the manner in which it was taught. Typically martial arts had been taught in a master-disciple manner, and were usually transmitted within family lines, often from father to son. Yang Luchan (1799–1872, Zheng's great grand-teacher) and his offspring marked the beginning of public teaching of taiji. Yang had been allowed to study within Chen family circles (where taijiquan was said to have originated), but soon began to see the merit of teaching publicly. As Yang was purported to have said in the late 1800s, taiji was not

> to challenge others but for self-defense, not to bully the world but to save the nation. . . . We are poor because we are weak; truly weakness is the cause of poverty. . . . the best method of saving the nation is to make saving the weak our highest priority. To ignore this is to be doomed to failure.[46]

By the early 1900s Yang's sons were participating in the newly formed "ecumenical" martial arts organizations in Beijing, and took the lead in offering taijiquan to the public.[47]

A natural evolution of styles of taijiquan took place. The influence of each practitioner's physique and abilities, as well as interests and goals, all left a mark on the actual taijiquan forms. By the 1900s, this resulted in at least a dozen substyles of taijiquan within both Chen and Yang family circles.[48] But more significantly, forms were modified to appeal to a wider audience. Yang's grandson, Yang Chengfu, modified their family form, taking out the more strenuous and martial moves specifically to reach a wider public.

Zheng Manqing and others of his generation, such as Chen Weiming, Dong Yingjie, and Xu Yusheng, continued the work of spreading and refining taijiquan study and teaching in public forums. They chose to place the "needs of the nation" above the "filial" demands of private lineages. Zheng himself felt that the keeping of secrets would ultimately diminish the art.

As Zheng matured in his own practice, he began to see the wisdom of his Yang predecessors in their promotion of taijiquan as a health exercise for the general populace. He knew from his own personal experience its profound health benefits and saw it as a means of improving his countrymen's health. As he later wrote:

> Without sound health, as without education, what good can one do to one's nation or social order, kith and kin, or neighbors? None at all![49]

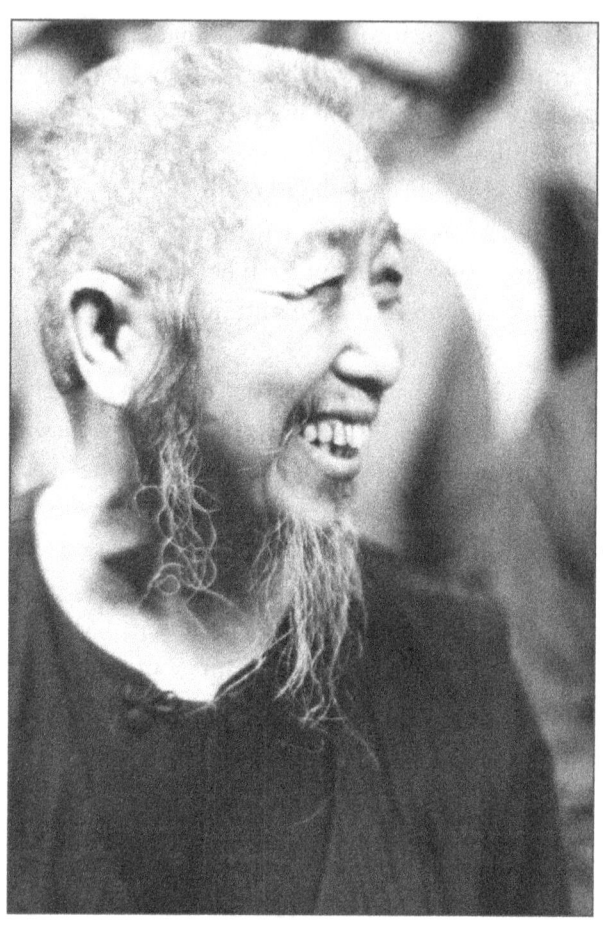

Zheng drew many followers,
not only because of his knowledge,
but also because of his warm personality.

Zheng saw how the Chinese people were suffering from sickness and poor self-esteem. Zheng felt that improved health and mind-set would help to "clear from us Chinese the undignified appellation of the 'infirm people of the Far East.'"[50] Thus, when Zheng writes that to withhold this gem was to ruin the country, or that on behalf of one's kin and country, one should study taijiquan, it should not be dismissed as a mere slogan.

Zheng's first dozen years of teaching took place during the upheaval of the Sino-Japanese War. It was clear to him that there were several problems inherent in the teaching and practice patterns of the past: the length of study needed to master taijiquan, the amount of time necessary for practice each day, and perseverance in study and practice.

As a result, over the next decade, Zheng Manqing decided to rework the Yang family taijiquan form because, citing national interests, he said, "I had to simplify the form in order to spread it, and I had to spread it so that it could make the people and the country strong."[51] By eliminating repeated moves he was able to condense the 128-move "long form" into a thirty-seven-move "short form." He felt this condensed form did not sacrifice the variety of moves nor adversely affect the potential quality of practice. This reduced the amount of time needed for a practice session from over a half hour to under ten minutes. He ultimately asserted, "I believe this book is in harmony with my teacher's [Yang Chengfu's] ideas,"[52] and received the support of his elder classmate Chen Weiming.

In his effort to popularize taijiquan practice, Zheng recommended ten minutes, morning and evening, of practice, rather than the hours of practice each day that were demanded in a traditional school. Zheng also cited other more practical reasons for doing taijiquan as opposed to other kinds of exercise: convenience, time, and low or no cost. It was safer than swimming and was not overly strenuous.[53]

Zheng also describes his internal struggle over what should or should not be shared openly. Could he follow the traditions of holding secrets back, potentially risking diminishing the art as well as the health of the country? No, he said. "If I also keep one secret or if I keep all of them, I would then be guilty of saving a pearl while my country went to ruin."[54] Yet he was nervous that he might be passing these secrets on to the wrong person. In the end, his desire to share the great benefits of taijiquan with the world won out.

It was in part because of potential health benefits that he felt taijiquan was particularly well suited for women. As a doctor of Chinese medicine, he applauded the emancipation of women from centuries of social and physical "restraints" (i.e., foot and breast binding and seclusion), and admonished that

> The health of a nation depends on the health of its women. Healthy mothers usually give birth to healthy babies while unhealthy mothers to unhealthy ones. Like sowing seeds, fertilized soil yields rich crops while barren soil poor ones. Since taking exercises is so important to women's health, it is most advisable for them to adopt taijiquan.[55]

He feared though that too much stimulation and activity would interfere with women's metabolism. He cited the traditional medical concept of women's health being based on "blood"[56] and that "blood being normally tranquil, so to speak, too strenuous activity for a woman will adversely affect her circulation."[57]

Beyond taijiquan's use as a health exercise, Zheng found in it one more vehicle for the teaching of the Confucian Dao. He was in a unique position to both add taijiquan to the repertoire of the gentleman-scholar, as well as to expand the reach of taijiquan ideas with an infusion of Chinese philosophy. Confucian, Daoist, and Neo-Confucian philosophy were important elements of his teachings of taijiquan. During a time when much of the writing on taijiquan focused on the physical aspects of practice, Zheng brought to his works fresh ideas from Mencius, the *Analects*, the *Yijing*, *The Art of War*, and the *Daodejing*, along with later philosophers such as Wang Yangming.

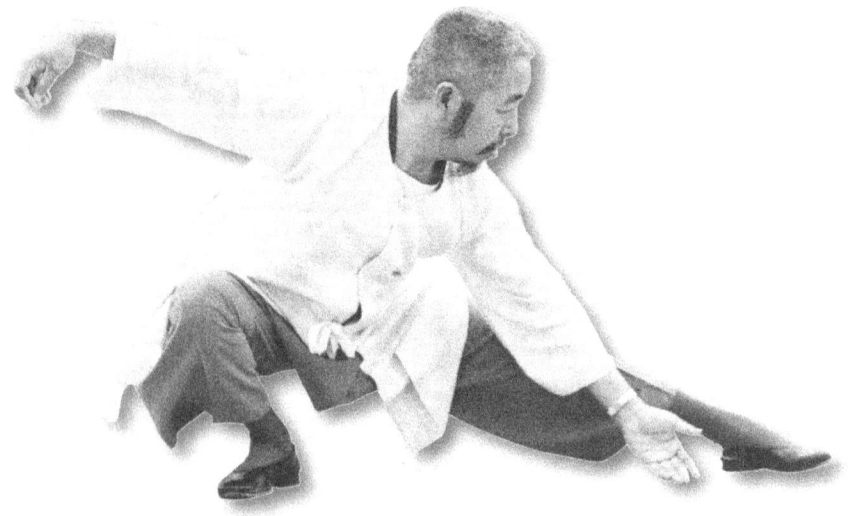

Photo courtesy of Robert W. Smith.

Conclusion

Zheng Manqing was a true Renaissance man who stepped beyond the bounds of traditional scholarship into the arena of martial arts. He brought with him the fruits of his previous studies, and in doing so, helped enrich taijiquan for people of all ages and nationalities. He incorporated into all of his work the ethics and philosophies of traditional China. Above all, Zheng Manqing, a man who indeed never tired of learning, was able to put into practice Confucius's words: "My Dao is that of an all-pervading unity."

Pinyin	Wade-Giles	Pinyin	Wade-Giles
Chen Weiming	Ch'en Wei-ming	Yang Luchan	Yang Lu-ch'an
Cai Yuanpei	Ts'ai Yuan-p'ei	Yongjia	Yung-chia
Ding Yidu	Ting I-tu	Zhang	Chang
Dong Yingjie	Tung Ying-chieh	Zhang Guang	Chang Kuang
Guang Wen	Kuang Wen	Zhejiang	Chekiang
Qian Mingshan	Ch'ien Ming-shan	Zheng Manqing	Cheng Man-ch'ing
Shizhong	Shih Chung, Shr Jung	Zheng Manran	Cheng Man-jan
Song You'an	Sung You-an	Zheng Qian	Cheng Ch'ien
Wenzhou	Wen-chou, Wen-chow	Zhi Rou	Chih Jou
Yang Chengfu	Yang Ch'eng-fu		

Notes

Many people have freely given ideas, information, and editorial assistance over the many years and versions of this article. I am deeply indebted to the many students of Zheng's with whom I have been able to associate through my years of taijiquan study and research work, as well as to classmates of mine who have shared an interest in exploring Zheng's life and works in depth. I would like specifically to thank Robert W. Smith for assistance on many details of Zheng's life; and from the University of Minnesota: Richard Mather (professor emeritus of Chinese) for help with Zheng's poetry, Romeyn Taylor (professor emeritus of Chinese history) for cogent criticism and encouragement, and Dr. Yuan Zhou and Yuh-shiow Wang (East Asian Library). Previous drafts have benefited from the feedback of historians Cynthia Brokaw, Jon Saari, and Ann Waltner, and anthropologist Margery Wolf. The late historian Angus MacDonald challenged me with some overarching questions at the beginning of this project, but passed away before seeing the fruits of his suggestions.

Biographical information for this article was drawn in the main from *Zheng Manqing's Memorial Book* [*Zhengzi ai si lu*], and an amplified English version of the same ("Cheng Tzu: Master of the Five Excellences" in *Full Circle*, 1: 2, 13–21). Other sources are indicated in the notes, which include autobiographical information from Zheng's numerous articles and books.

Western dates are used in this article. Every effort has been made to corroborate dates as accurately as possible; however, there are occasions where information available does not yield a clear timeline (also see note number 2). For consistency's sake, Pinyin romanization is used for transliteration of Chinese, including quoted material, except for names more familiar in other forms and published works that use other systems. Translations are my own unless otherwise indicated.

This article was presented in slightly different forms for the Midwest Council for Asian Affairs (1991) for a master's degree paper in the Department of East Asian Studies, University of Minnesota.

Abbreviations
Simplified Methods *T'ai Chi Ch'uan: A Simplified Method for Health and Self-Defense.*
Thirteen Treatises *Cheng Tzu's Thirteen Treatises on T'ai Chi Ch'uan.*
Chinese Painting *Traditional Chinese Paintings of the Southern School: Works by Man-jan Cheng.*
ZGJXD *Zhongguo jinxiandai renwu minghao da cidian.*

1. *Analects of Confucius*, book 4, chapter 15.
2. Zheng's Chinese birth date is Guangxu 28th year, 25th day of the 6th moon. I have arrived at the Western date by consulting the standard reference, *Liangqian nianlai zhongxi li duizhao biao* [Comparative Table of Chinese-Western Calendars for Two Thousand Years, Beijing: Sanlian Publishing, 1956]. There are a fair number of discrepancies between dates or ages in various material on Zheng. This may be attributed to confusion between different methods of calculating ages (one is considered to be one year old at birth, and another year is added at New Year's) and translation between the traditional and Western dating systems. Thus all ages given for Zheng (within this article as well as other people's material) should be taken as accurate within two years.
3. One's given name would have been used within the family, or by teachers, and a *zi*, or style name, was taken at twenty. It was common, particularly among the educated and artistic, to use alternate names, such as pen names, nicknames, and studio names. For well-known people such as Zheng and many of his associates, these names can be found in special indexes (e.g., ZGJXD).
4. These names will be found on his paintings, calligraphy works, and books, in signature and chop. Hermit of the Jade Well was one of his most commonly used appellations, which he used from at least the late 1940s on.
5. Throughout China's thousands of years of organized governance, place-names have changed, often back and forth between two names, as in the case of Yongia (Yung-chia) and Wenzhou (Wen-chou or Wenchow). Geographical dictionaries, gazetteers, and historical maps can be consulted for these changes.
6. *Manran san lun*, p. 9.
7. According to one source, Zheng's family had been wealthy in previous generations, but a fire had destroyed their property (Su Shaoqing "Wujue laoren," p. 6).
8. It is customary for a woman to maintain her own family name even after

marriage. Her offspring would bear her husband's surname.
9. *Manran san lun*, p. 9. The Tang dynasty (618–905) was one of the richest periods in Chinese poetry, producing such famous poets as Du Fu, Li Bai, and Wang Wei. Their poems are memorized in school and are used as models for writing.
10. In her later years, Zhang Guang (c. 1878–1970) used the style name Old Lady Redfern (*Hongwei Laoren*) and, in her earlier years, Virtue Harmony (*De Yi*). Zhang specialized in the "birds and flowers" genre of painting. She worked at a number of jobs, including as principal of a teachers' training school and as a professor of art in Shanghai, Beijing, Hangzhou, and Guangdong (ZGJXD entry no. 4702). The "outline style" of painting, also called "detailed brush" (*gongbi*), uses carefully executed fine outlines that are then filled with color.
11. Wang's given name was Ruyüan. He lived from 1867 to 1923 and was from Longxiang, Zhejiang Province. His style name was Xiangchan (also written as Xiangquan). His studio was named Fragrant Leaf (*Xiangye Lou*). He was an expert at flower and plant paintings and landscapes and had many disciples, the young Zheng among them (ZGJXD entry no. 4303).
12. Xieyi literally means "writing the thoughts." It is a very fluid, expressive style that demands great mastery of the brush, ink, and paper.
13. Cai Yuanpei (Ts'ai Yuan-p'ei, 1868–1940) was one of the most influential educators of early Republican China. He was educated within the traditional system and passed the highest exam (*jinshi*, received scholar) at the very young age of twenty-two. Cai served as minister of education, chancellor of Beijing University, and was founder and president of the Academia Sinica, the national research institute. In his work he sought a synthesis of Chinese and Western intellectual processes. Cai supported the practice of taijiquan and wrote prefaces for a number of taijiquan books, including those by Yang Chengfu (1933) and Xu Longhou (1921).
14. This early album appears to be the same as one entitled *Zheng Manqing xiesheng jiapin* [Zheng Manqing's paintings from life], dated 1924, which is reproduced in *Zheng Manqing huaji*, plates 31–34. Among the well-known people who wrote calligraphic inscriptions for it (dated 1926) was Cai Yuanpei.
15. Ben Lo, one of Zheng's senior students, reports that Zheng did not study Shaolin boxing, but rather "internal exercises" for qi cultivation such as baduanjin. *Shaolin gongfu* refers to a wide range of popular exercises that were associated with Shaolin Temple traditions (Ben Lo interview, September 1995). In a similar fashion nowadays, these kinds of exercises are often associated with *qigong* practices.
16. Chen established the society in 1925, after eight years of study with Yang. It is not clear from material consulted whether Yang moved to Shanghai or was

visiting and teaching on a regular basis (see Chen, *Taijiquan dawen*).

[17] There is some confusion about the precise dates of Zheng's study with Yang Chengfu. Some sources (e.g., *Zheng Manqing xiansheng aisi lu*, p. 4) state that Zheng began with Yang at twenty-seven *sui* (approximately twenty-five to twenty-six years of age in the Western dating method), which would be around 1927. However, Zheng himself wrote in his preface to Yang's 1934 book, *Taijiquan tiyong quan shu*, that he was introduced to Yang in *Renshan zhengyue* (February 1932) by a Mr. Po Qiucheng. That would place Zheng's period of study with Yang from 1932 until 1936, when Yang passed away. Chen Weiming's calligraphed preface (dated 1947) to Zheng's *Thirteen Treatises*, p. 1, states that Zheng studied with Yang for six years.

[18] See R. Smith, (1995). "Zheng Manqing and Taijiquan: A Clarification of Role." *Journal of Asian Martial Arts*, 4(1), 52–53.

[19] Zheng was studying both with Qian and Yang during the same period. Qian Mingshan (c.1875–c.1944) had the given name of Qian Zhenhuang. He was from Yanghu (today's Changzhou), Jiangsu Province. He passed the jinshi examination in 1904 and, after leaving work in the government, became known as a scholar and calligrapher (ZGJXD no. 7642).

[20] It is generally considered that Yang was not literate, or not literate enough to write the books that appeared under his name. His first book, *Taijiquan shi yongfa*, is said to have been ghostwritten by another senior student, Dong Yingie, in 1931. Additionally, Chen Weiming wrote three books under his own name (*Taijiquan shu*, *Taijiquan hen*, and *Taiji jian*), though in each of these books he mentions that he was recording Yang Chengfu's words. (See Wile, *T'ai-chi Touchstones*, p. iii–iv.)

[21] This book is translated in full in Lo and Inn's *Cheng-tzu's Thirteen Treatises*. It was completed in 1947 and published in 1950 after Zheng moved to Taiwan. Yu's inscription is dated November 1948. Chen's preface is dated April 1947.

[22] When Zheng departed for the United States, the association was left in the hands of his senior student, Liu Xihong. It is currently headed by Xu Yizhong. *Shizhong* is a philosophical term meaning "at the right time." (The Taiwan group romanized the term as *Shih Chung*, the American group as *Shr Jung*.) Information on the Taiwan Shizhong group is culled from Smith, *Chinese Boxing*; Smalheiser, "Push Hands . . ." (interview with Abraham Liu); *Taijiquan zazhi*; and Ben Lo (interviews, August and September 1995).

[23] "De jia shu," from *Yujing caotang shi xuji*, vol. 2, p. 4. In *Manran san lun*, Zheng indicates that he was the youngest of six children (p. 3). This reference to a younger brother may be poetic license, or may refer to the youngest of his elder brothers. Zheng may also have been simplifying the reference so as to fit the

poetic meter.

24 It was arranged for Zheng to use the Columbia University Library. For a writer or researcher, the open stacks at the library would have been a great temptation, especially as compared with the closed-stack system common to Chinese libraries (Ben Lo, interview, August 1995). In appreciation, Zheng donated copies of some of his works to a number of university libraries across the United States.

25 *Thirteen Treatises*, p. 108–109.

26 Information on the New York Shizhong school is culled from discussions with Zheng's students between 1979 and 1994, including Ed Young, Maggie Newman, Lori Reinstein, Ken Van Sickle, Jane Faigao, Bataan Faigao, Carol Yamasaki, and Wolfe Lowenthal, and from numerous articles in *Full Circle* and *T'ai Chi Player*.

27 This is an overarching theme in his book *Renwen qianshuo*.

28 Zheng Manqing was not the first Chinese person to be interested in promoting Chinese ideals to foreigners and overseas Chinese. In 1895 reformer and Confucian follower Kang Youwei (1858–1927) had suggested in a memorial to the Qing emperor that not only should Confucianism continue to be spread among the Chinese, but that Confucian academies should even be set up overseas. See Spence, *Gates of Heavenly Peace*, p. 42.

29 Ed Young, "Character Study," p. 3.

30 *Chinese Paintings*, p. 2.

31 *Chinese Paintings*, p. 20.

32 From the painting *Green Mountain*, in *Chinese Paintings*, plate 6, dated 1973, with my editing.

33 *Manran san lun*, p. 72–73.

34 See Zheng's *Renwen qianshuo*, author's introduction, ch. 39, "The Cultural Renaissance"; as well as Anon., "Principles for the Promotion of the Chinese Cultural Renaissance Movement"; and Uhalley, "Taiwan's Response to the Cultural Revolution."

35 See *Renwen qianshuo*, author's introduction.

36 Among Zheng's publishers were such well-respected presses as the Commercial Press, Zhonghua Shuju, and the National Palace Museum. He also self-published a number of books, a common custom among Chinese scholars.

37 *Manran san lun*, p. 2. Both Wang Wei (699–759) and Guang Wen (fl. 742–755) flourished during the culturally rich Tian Bao reign period (742–755) of the Emperor Xuanzong in the early Tang dynasty. Wang Wei is credited with having founded a style of painting called *pomo* (broken ink) that spawned the more expressive ink painting styles popular in scholarly and amateur circles. Guang

Wen, whose actual name was Zheng Qian, served in the Tang court as assistant chief musician and later as head of the *Guanwen guan*, the Office of Director of Studies. Zheng presented one of his paintings to Emperor Xuanzong, who was a great patron of the arts. The emperor inscribed the painting with "Three Excellences Zheng Qian," referring to Zheng's skill at painting, poetry, and calligraphy. After a while, Zheng became known in learned circles as Zheng Guang Wen, which literally means "Broadly Learned Zheng" (see *Xin tang shu juan* 202, p. 5766–5767, by Ouyang Xiu, Beijing: Zhonghua shuju, 1975). Zheng Manqing admired Zheng Qian's breadth of learning and carved a seal in admiration that he used occasionally on his artwork. The seal bore the inscription "Born 1,200 Years after Guang Wen" (see e.g., *Zheng Manqing xian-sheng shuhua tezhan mulu*, pl. 15).

38 *Manran san lun*, p. 2.

39 *Manran san lun*, p. 44. The dantian, or "field of cinnabar," is an important energy point in the body, located a couple of inches below and internal to the navel.

40 *Yiquan*, author's introduction, p. 3.

41 The six senior students were Tam Gibbs, Ed Young, Maggie Newman, Lou Kleinsmith, Mort Raphael, and Stanley Israel.

42 "In the morning hearing the Dao, in the evening die without regret" (in James Legge, *Confucian Analects*, bk. 4, ch. 8). Confucius also said, "If some years were added to my life, I would give fifty to the study of the *Yi[jing]*, and then I might come to be without great faults" (*Analects*, bk. 7, ch. 16, Legge).

43 These are among the material in *Zhengzi ai si lu*.

44 *Zheng Manqing xiansheng shuhua tezhan mulu* [Catalogue of Mr. Zheng Manqing's special exhibit of calligraphy and painting] p. 1–3.

45 Zheng is now listed, for example, in mainland-published martial arts biographies and bibliographies such as the *Zhongguo wushu da cidian* [Dictionary of Chinese martial arts, p. 489, p. 504], in Yang lineage charts found in martial arts books, as well as the *ZGJXD*.

46 Wile, *T'ai-chi Touchstones*, p. x. This is not to suggest that the educated men who took up taijiquan were not able to fight. Zheng himself took on many challengers. See Smith, *Chinese Boxing*, p. 25–46.

47 Wile, *T'ai-chi Touchstones*, p. 153. These are supposed to be Yang Luchan's words as spoken to Yang Chengfu. As Yang Luchan was already dead before Yang Chengfu was born, we could speculate that these words may actually reflect Yang Chengfu's attitudes, and were being purposely antedated (as is common practice in China) to make a point with more authority.

48 For more on the history of taijiquan, see Draeger and Smith, *Asian Fighting Arts*,

p. 35–39, and DeMarco, "The Origin and Evolution of Taijiquan."
[49] *Simplified Method*, pp. 26–27.
[50] *Simplified Method*, p. 57.
[51] *Thirteen Treatises*, p. 104.
[52] *Thirteen Treatises*, p. 108.
[53] *Simplified Method*, p. 52.
[54] *Thirteen Treatises*, p. 87.
[55] *Simplified Method*, p. 54.
[56] In traditional Chinese medicine, "blood" (*xue*) incorporates more than the Western physical blood. It provides nourishment, maintenance, and moisture through the body, moving through the blood vessels and meridians. It is moved by the qi of the heart and chest. See Kaptchuk, *The Web That Has No Weaver*, p. 201.
[57] *Simplified Method*, p. 53.

Bibliography
Works by Zheng Manqing
(Zheng Manran, Cheng Man-ching, Cheng Man-jan)

Books

Note: Zheng's taijiquan writings can be divided into five "books," which have been published in varying combinations in both Chinese and English editions, noted as follows:

- *Zhengzi taijiquan shisan pian* [Thirteen treatises] Section 1
- *Zhengzi taijiquan shisan pian* [Thirteen treatises] Section 2
- *Zhengzi taijiquan zixiu xinfa* [New method]
- *T'ai Chi Ch'uan: A Simplified Method* (in English)
- *T'ai Chi* (in English)

Cheng, M., & Smith, R. (1967). *T'ai chi*. Rutland, VT: Charles E. Tuttle Co.
Gibbs, T. (Trans.). (1981). *Lao-tzu: My words are very easy to understand*. Berkeley: North Atlantic Books. [Translation of *Laozi yizhi jie*.]
Lo, B., & Inn, M. (Trans.). (1985). *Cheng Tzu's thirteen chapters on t'ai chi ch'uan*. Berkeley: North Atlantic Books. [Authorized translation of *Zhengzi taijiquan shisan pian*, sections 1 and 2.]
Tseng, B. (Trans.). (1981). *T'ai chi ch'uan: A simplified method of calisthenics for health and self-defense*. Berkeley: North Atlantic Books.
Wile, D. (Trans.). (1983). *Master Cheng's thirteen chapters on t'ai chi ch'uan*. Brook-

lyn: Sweet Ch'i Press. [Translation of *Zhengzi taijiquan shisan pian*, section 1.]

Wile, D. (Trans.). (1985). *Cheng Man-ch'ing's advanced t'ai chi form instructions*. Brooklyn: Sweet Ch'i Press. [Translation of *Zhengzi taijiquan shisan pian*, section 2 and additional material.]

Zheng, M. (n.d.). *Guke jingwei* [Subtleties of orthopedics]. Text not extant.

Zheng, M. (n.d.). *Tang shi zhen du* [Probing and measuring Tang poetry]. Taiwan: n.p.

Zheng, M. (n.d.). *Manqing zixuan* [Manqing freestyle poetry]. Text not extant.

Zheng, M. (n.d.). *Yujing caotang shiji* [Jade well grass hall poetry collection]. Vol. 1. Taibei: self-published. [c. 1961].

Zheng, M. (1950). *Zhengzi taijiquan shisan pian* [Master Zheng's thirteen treatises on taijiquan] Sections 1 and 2. Taibei: n.p.

Zheng, M. (1961). *Nuke xinfa* [Essence of gynecology]. Taibei: National Traditional Chinese Medical Research Institute.

Zheng, M. (1962). *T'ai chi ch'uan: A simplified method of calisthenics for health and self-defense*. Taibei: Shih Chung T'ai-chi Chuan Center.

Zheng, M. (1965). *Zhengzi taijiquan zixiu xinfa* [Master Zheng's new method of taijiquan self-cultivation]. Taibei: Shizhong quanshe. [Includes *Zhengzi taijiquan shisan pian*, section 1]. Reprinted 1977.

Zheng, M. (1966). *Tan ai ba yao* [Eight important points on cancer]. Taibei: Guoli zhongguo yi yao yanjiu suo. Pamphlet.

Zheng, M. (1971). *Laozi yizhi jie* [*Lao-Tzu: My words are very easy to understand*]. Taibei: Zhonghua shuju.

Zheng, M. (1971). *Lunyu shizhi* [Explanation of the meaning of the *Analects*]. Taibei: Zhonghua shuju.

Zheng, M. (1971). *Xueyong xinjie* [New commentary on *Great learning* and *Doctrine of the mean*]. Taibei: Commercial Press.

Zheng, M. (1971). *Yujing caotang shiji* [Jade well grass hall poetry collection], Vol. 2. Taibei: self-published.

Zheng, M. (1973). *Renwen qianshuo* [A simplified explanation of man and his culture]. Taiwan: self-published.

Zheng, M. (1974). *Manran san lun* [Three treatises of Manran]. Taibei: Zhonghua shuju.

Zheng, M. (1974). *Yiquan* [The complete *Book of changes*]. Taibei: Meiya Publishing.

Articles

Gibbs, T., & Young, E. (Trans.). (Fall 1983). The Professor lectures. *T'ai chi player*,

1, 1–2. [First introductory lecture on *zhongyong*.]

Gibbs, T. (Trans.). (Dec. 1986). Professor Cheng on self defense. *T'ai chi player*, 4.

Hennessy, M. (Trans.). (1971). *The story of strong man (Qiangren zhuan)*. Manuscript. [Autobiographical essay.]

Hennessy, M. (Trans.). (1988). *Principles for living*. Manuscript, 3pp.

Hennessy, M. (Trans.). (1989). *Cheng Man-ch'ing's last statement concerning t'ai chi ch'uan*. Manuscript, 2pp. [Signed "Man-jan, Spring Day, 1975."]

Hennessy, M. (1995). *Cheng Man-ch'ing: Master of Five Excellences*. Berkeley: Frog.

Zheng, M. (n.d.). *Xingben lun* [Discussion of man's original nature]. [Appendix to *Xueyong xinjie*.]

Zheng, M. (June 10, 1968). Meditation corresponds perfectly with medical principles; It is the bridge to better health and the path to longer life. *Zhongyang ribao*. [In *Cheng Man-ch'ing's advanced form instructions*, 121–125.]

Zheng, M. (July 20, 1970). *Principles of wisdom in taijiquan*. Taijiquan yanjiusuo.

Zheng, M. (July 20, 1971). A glimpse at the fifth anniversary of the Taijiquan Research Association. *Taijiquan yanjiu suo*.

Zheng, M. (Dec. 16, 1974). Man tan wuchin xi zhi xiong jing [An explanation of the constant bear movement from the five animals]. *Changliu*. Taibei: Taiwan Railway Bureau. Revised ed. *Taijiquan zazhi*, April 1983.

Zheng, M. (July 1984). Professor Cheng on the chung-yung. *T'ai chi player*, 1–3.

Zheng, M. (April 1984). Taijiquan yu tiyu [Taijiquan and physical education]. *Taijiquan zazhi*, 10–14.

Zheng, M. (July 1985). Professor Cheng on the chung-yung. *T'ai chi player*, 1–2.

Lectures

Gibbs, T., & Young, E. (Trans.). (Jan. 1974). Professor Cheng's health lecture. Manuscript, 11 pp. [New York City.]

Zheng, M. *Zhongyong (Doctrine of the Mean)*. Lecture series for Shizhong Center, New York City. See under "articles" and "secondary sources".

Zheng, M. (June 20, 1971). *Kongzi yu Laozi zhi yitong* [Similarities and differences between Confucius and Laozi]. Taibei: Ministry of Education, Department of Culture. [Pamphlet.]

Zheng, M. (April 1984). Tan taijiquan [Speaking about taijiquan]. *Taijiquan zazhi*, 32, 6–7. [Feb. 26, 1975, at Miaoli Detective Bureau Hall.]

Painting Collections and Calligraphy

(1926). *Zheng Manqing xiesheng jiapin* [High quality paintings from life by Zheng Manqing], or *Zheng Manqing huace* [Painting album by Zheng Manqing]. [Reproduced in *Zheng Manran shuhua ji*, 31–34.]

(1961). *The art of Cheng Man-ch'ing* [Manran xieyi]. Taibei: Heritage Press.

(1971). *Zheng Manran shuhua ji* [Collection of Zheng Manran's calligraphy and painting]. Taibei: Zhonghua shuju. [Catalogue of exhibit at Taibei Provincial Museum.]

(1973). *Traditional Chinese paintings of the southern school: Works by Man-jan Cheng.* Yonkers: Hudson River Museum.

(1982). *Zheng Manqing xiansheng shuhua tezhan mulu* [Special exhibition of painting and calligraphic works by Mr. Zheng Manqing]. Taibei: National Palace Museum. [Reprinted from *The art of Cheng Man-ch'ing*.]

Movies

Yang style t'ai chi ch'uan. Produced by Shr Jung Cultural Center. Color. Narrative, form, push-hands, sword, approx. 20 min.

Untitled. Taijiquan form and pushing hands. New York City. B&W, approx. 10 min.

Untitled. Taijiquan demonstration. Taiwan. B&W, approx. 10 min.

Secondary Sources

Anon. (Oct. 29, 1973). Hold it! *New Yorker*, 35–36.

Anon. (Dec. 10, 1974). The brush. *New Yorker*, 41.

Anon. (1975). *Zheng Manqing xiansheng ai si lu* [Mr. Zheng Manqing's funeral and memorial book]. Taibei: n.p.

Anon. (April 25, 1975). Cheng Man-ching is dead at 73; Calligrapher, painter and poet. *New York Times*, 32.

Chen, W. (n.d.). *Taijiquan shu* [The art of taijiquan]. Hong Kong: Wushu chubanshe.

Chen, W. (1929). *Taijiquan hen* [Questions and answers on taijiquan]. Shanghai: n.p. [Reprint, Taibei: Zhongguo taijiquan xue shu yanjiuhui, 1967.]

DeMarco, M. (1992). The origin and evolution of taijiquan. *Journal of Asian martial arts, 1*(1), 8–25.

Dong, Y. (1975). *Taijiquan shiyi* [Principles of taijiquan]. Hong Kong: Zhonghua shuju.

Draeger, D., & Smith, R. (1974). *Asian fighting arts*. New York: Berkeley Medallion.

Faigo, B. (1984). Here it is: A conversational portrait. *Full circle, 1*:1, 2–12.

Gibbs, T. (1984). Tam Gibbs' notes from Prof. Cheng's class. *T'ai chi player, 2,* 5.

Gibbs, T. (Trans.). (1985). Cheng Tzu: Master of the five excellences. *Full circle, 1*:2, 13–20. [English rendition with Madame Zheng.]

Hennessy, M. (n.d.). Translation and commentary on Cheng Man-ch'ing's "principles for living." Manuscript. 3pp.

Lad, J. (1983). What does it mean to say that t'ai-chi ch'uan is scientific? *T'ai chi player, 1*, 6–8.

Lad, J. (1984). On mobilization of ch'i: Activating a mechanism or giving a signal? *T'ai ch'i player, 2*, 6–8.

Lerhman, F. (1975). Untitled. *Shr Jung newsletter, 1*:1, 7. [In memory of Professor Cheng.]

Lo, B., & Smith, R. (Trans.). (1985). *T'ai chi ch'uan ta-wen* [Questions and answers on taijiquan]. Berkeley: North Atlantic Books.

Lo, P. (1985). Zuojia taijiquan shiyi [Settling the uncertainties about Zuo family taijiquan]. *Taijiquan zazhi, 40*, 8–14.

Lo, P., et al. (1979). *The essence of t'ai chi ch'uan*. Berkeley: North Atlantic Books.

Lowenthal, W. (1983). The wonder of t'ai-chi ch'uan. *T'ai chi player, 1*, 2–3.

Lowenthal, W. (1984). The virtue of t'ai-chi ch'uan. *T'ai chi player, 2*, 5–6.

Lowenthal, W. (1985). The negative aspect of t'ai-chi ch'uan. *T'ai chi player, 3*, 10–11.

Lowenthal, W. (1991). *There are no secrets: Professor Cheng Man-ch'ing's t'ai chi ch'uan*. Berkeley: North Atlantic Books.

Lowenthal, W. (1994). *Gateway to the miraculous: Further explorations in the Tao of Cheng Man-ch'ing*. Berkeley: Frog.

Mu, B. (n.d.). Wujuede shuhuajia Zheng Manqing [Painter-calligrapher of five excellences Zheng Manqing]. *Taijiquan zazhi, 25*, 6.

Smalheiser, M. (1990). Push hands is a game of skill. *T'ai Chi, 145*. [Interview with Abraham Liu.]

Smith, R. (1974). *Chinese boxing: Masters and methods*. Tokyo: Kodansha.

Smith, R. (1975). A Master Passes. *Shr Jung newsletter, 1*:1, 2–7.

Smith, R. (1984). A defense of Cheng Man-ch'ing. *Inside kung-fu, 11*:2, 6. [Letter to the editor.]

Smith, R. (1995). Zheng Manqing and taijiquan: A clarification of role. *Journal of Asian martial arts, 4*(1), 50–65.

Su, S. (April 1983). Wujue laoren: Zheng Manqing gong xiao zhuan [Old man of five excellences: A short biography of Zheng Manqing]. *Taijiquan zazhi*, 6–7.

Wile, D. (1983). *T'ai chi touchstones: Yang family secret transmissions*. Brooklyn: Sweet Ch'i Press.

Xu, L. (Xu Yusheng). (1982). *Taijiquan shi tujie* [Illustrated explanation of taijiquan]. Taibei: Hualian chubanshe.

Xu, Y. (April 1983). Dao'en shi, zhi yishi [Mourning our beloved teacher, some anecdotes]. *Taijiquan zazhi*, 8.

Yamasaki, C. (1986). Notes from Professor Cheng's class. *T'ai chi player, 3*, 4–5.

Yang C. (1983). *Taijiquan tiyong quan shu* [Complete book of substance and application of taijiquan]. Taibei: Laogu wenhua shiye.

Yang C., et al. (1984). *Taijiquan xuanbian*. Beijing: Beijingshi Zhongguo shudian.

Young, E. (July 1985). Some notes on translation. *T'ai chi player*, 3.

Xinhua Press. (1992). *Zhongguo jinxiandai renwu minghao dacidian* [Dictionary of alternate names of modern Chinese personages]. Zhejiang: Xinhua Press.

Background Material

Chang, E., & Etzold, T. (Eds.). (1976). *China in the 1920s: Nationalism and revolution*. New York: New Viewpoints.

Dennerline, J. (1988). *Qian Mu and the world of seven mansions*. New Haven: Yale University Press.

Furth, C. (1976). *The limits of change*. Cambridge: Harvard University Press.

Kaptchuk, T. (1983). *The web that has no weaver*. New York: Congdon and Weed.

Legge, J., (Trans.). (1971). *The Analects, Confucius*. New York: Dover.

Liu, F. (1956). *A military history of modern China 1924–1945*. Princeton: Princeton University Press.

Lowe, H. (1983). *The adventures of Wu*. Princeton: Princeton University Press.

Rankin, M. (1986). *Elite activism and political transformation in China: Zhejiang province, 1865–1911*. Stanford: Stanford University Press.

Saari, J. (1990). *Legacies of childhood: Growing up Chinese in a time of crisis, 1890–1920*. Cambridge: Council on East Asian Studies, Harvard University.

Shieh, M. (1970). *The Kuomintang: Selected historical documents, 1894–1969*. New York: St. John's University Press.

Smith, R. (1983). *China's cultural heritage: The Ch'ing dynasty, 1644–1912*. Boulder: Westview Press.

Spence, J. (1982). *Gates of heavenly peace*. New York: Penguin Books.

Spence, J. (1990). *In search of modern China*. New York: Norton.

Schwarcz, V. (1986). *The Chinese enlightenment*. Berkeley: University of California.

Taylor, R. (1990). *Religious dimensions of Confucianism*. Albany: State University of New York Press.

Uhalley, S. (1967). Taiwan's response to the Cultural Revolution. *Asia Survey*, VII, 824–829.

Wolf, M. (1991). *Thrice-told tale: Feminism, postmodernism, and ethnographic responsibility*. Stanford: Stanford University Press.

The Development of Zheng Manqing Taijiquan in Malaysia
by Nigel Sutton, M.A.

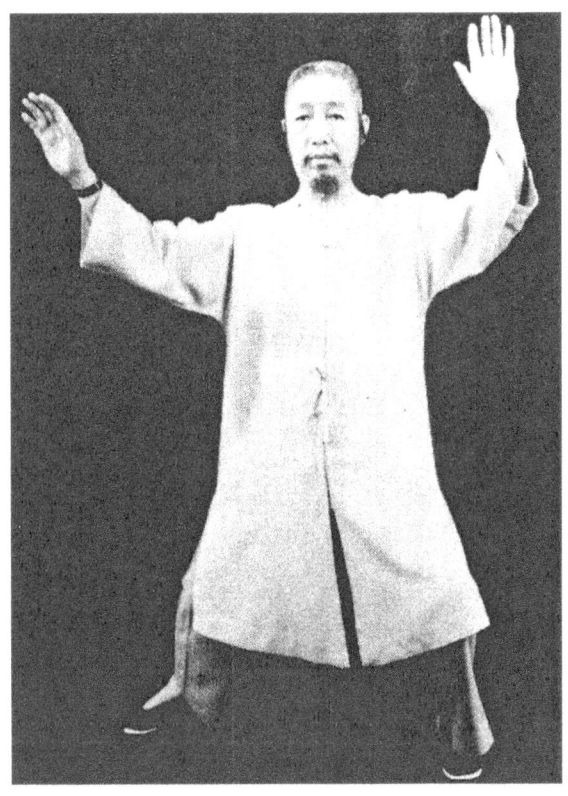

Zheng Manqing moving into embrace-tiger posture.
All illustrations courtesy of Charles E. Tuttle Co.

Most authorities on taijiquan acknowledge the development and existence of five main schools that have come into being as distinct entities during the later part of the twentieth century and the early part of this century. It may be argued, however, that the style most responsible for the enormous growth of awareness and practice of the art on the world stage is that which in Asia is referred to as the Zheng style, after its founder, Zheng Manqing. While the founder always acknowledged the Yang style origins of his art, his teacher being Yang Chengfu, as time passed and Zheng applied his experience in other related fields to his teaching of taijiquan, it became apparent his art had grown into a distinct style in its own right.

In order to understand the art of Zheng Manqing, it is essential to know something about the man himself. A staunch traditionalist, professor of art, renowned calligrapher, and accomplished doctor of Chinese medicine, Zheng was also an innovator and was thus forced to live on that knife edge, peculiar to Oriental cultures, where demand for the observance of long-established tradition must be weighed against the necessity for innovation and progress. That this state of dynamic tension was of concern to Zheng is illustrated by the reference he made to it in his writings. In essay number 6 of book 3 of his *Manran san lun*, Zheng talks about "understanding change," detailing when change should occur. Although ostensibly writing about painting, everything he writes may be applied to taijiquan. In essay number 8, entitled "Reckoning Mastery," his comments may also be directly applied to his experience of taijiquan (Wile, 1985).

Although in his writings on taijiquan Zheng always named Yang Chengfu as the source of his knowledge, in an article on the development of power in calligraphy he revealed the important role of the Zuo Laipeng system of internal strength training in the growth of his own skill and in his understanding of the art (Wile, 1985: 148). Indeed, it is generally recognized by practitioners of the Zheng style that it was the injection of the core elements of the Zuo system into his thirty-seven-posture form that made his system unique.

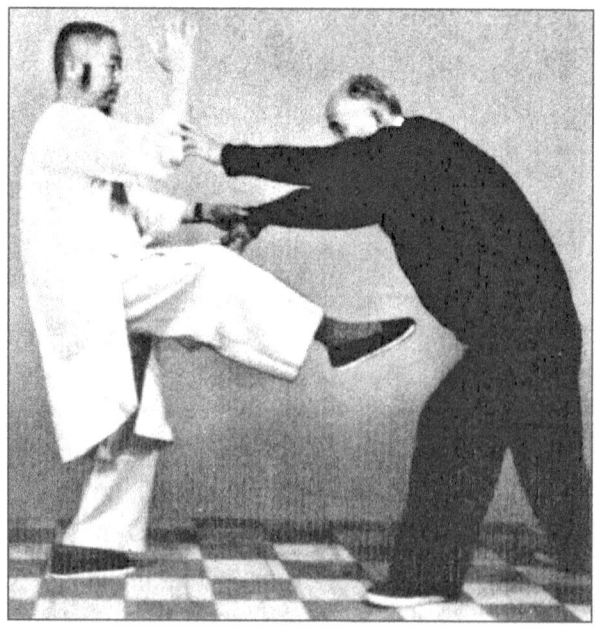

Zheng with T. T. Liang Tongcai.
An application of golden cock stands on one leg.

The thirty-seven postures themselves are based closely, if only superficially, on the Yang-style form, and Zheng gave as his reasons for shortening the traditional form a combination of personal impatience and laziness, as well as the demand for a shorter period of study if the art were to be popularized.

In order to understand the essence of Zheng's form, we have to look beyond this smoke screen to see that the emphasis is on principle rather than technique, and so contained within the form are all the movement principles that may be found in the traditional form but without so many repetitions of particular movements. So while it may not contain such moves as fan through back, needle at sea bottom, or part the horse's mane, the principles these postures embody may be found in fair lady plays shuttles, planting punch, and left and right ward-off respectively.

What exactly the Zuo system consists of is a source of contention among Zheng's students, and this I will examine later, when discussing the style's practice in Malaysia. Suffice it to say that at this stage it places a greater emphasis on *song* (Wile, 1985: 148), taijiquan's state of alert relaxation, than does the Yang style.

There is much disagreement, even among Zheng's long-term disciples, as to his personal training history, and probably the closest we come to a definitive version is given in his obituary/biography.[1] It is stated there that in his youth Zheng studied Shaolin boxing but later took up taijiquan for the sake of his health. One cryptic sentence alludes to his studies with Zhang Qingling, from whom he learned the Zuo method. That Zhang was his martial arts elder brother in the Yang family tradition caused some difficulties in that Zheng could not openly refer to him as his teacher.

Song Zijian, one of Zheng's oldest surviving students in Taiwan, asserts that Zheng was sent to Zhang Qingling to learn push-hands, armed with a letter of introduction from his teacher Yang Chengfu. The particular approach to push-hands he was to learn from Zhang Qingling was *song rou* push-hands, which may literally be translated as "relaxed and soft," both of which are hallmarks of the Zuo system and were to become the same for the Zheng system.[2]

While Zheng himself was always passionately interested in the martial aspects of the art, in attempting to popularize it he stressed those aspects he felt legitimized the art, both as the pursuit of a learned gentleman and of a person seeking the widest range of benefits. Because of his medical background and his own experience of being cured of tuberculosis through practice, he stressed the art's strengthening and curative aspects.

As a student of Chinese philosophy, the relationship of the *Yijing* and the *Daodejing* to the philosophical foundation of the art were of great importance to him. Additionally, as a practitioner of the fine arts, both the aesthetic qualities and the striving for perfection of form were of great concern to Zheng's development and approach to taijiquan.

The most obvious changes Zheng made, other than shortening the form, were softening and relaxing the postures, so some exponents of the Yang style accuse Zheng stylists of doing "old man's taijiquan." It would be a mistake, however, to assume this external appearance of ease means the postures themselves are effortless. Because of the required degree of profound relaxation, a great strain is placed on the supporting leg, so what in Yang style is often described as being a 70-30 stance becomes a 99.9-0.1 stance, the numbers describing the percentage of weight on each leg. The aim is "to borrow the strength of the earth and the qi of the heavens," which means, in terms of form, the legs do the work while the upper body is kept as empty and relaxed as possible.

In form practice, Zheng emphasized adherence to principle rather than an overemphasis on the techniques represented by individual postures. In Zheng style the purpose of form is to teach the basic principles such as sinking, relaxation, and the constant interchange of yin and yang, as found in the changes from substantial to insubstantial and then back again.

As well as shortening the form, Zheng only emphasized one of the three traditional taiji weapons, the straight sword, because it most exemplifies and embodies the principles of the art. Zheng also introduced the sword sticking exercises that are another hallmark of his style. In this freestyle exercise, the practitioners keep their sword blades in contact as they maneuver, attempting to attack their opponent without losing the connection. This exercise is a logical extension of push-hands and is particularly effective for training *ting jing*, or sensitivity. In addition, Zheng emphasized a range of auxiliary exercises for the development of *neigong* (internal strength). These exercises are widely regarded as elements of the Zuo Laipeng system.

The exact date when Zheng Manqing first devised the thirty-seven-posture form is unclear, although in his writings he stated that he first taught it in 1937 in Henan Province (Wile, 1985: 192). Song Zijian also remembers it as first being taught then, although he stated that Zheng only had six or seven students at the time.[3] Chia Siewpang, who studied with Zheng in China, relates that he learned the form from him in 1936 (Chia, 1983).

When he went to Taiwan in 1949, Zheng's government connections and in particular his relationship with Chiang Kai-shek's wife, to whom he was a personal art tutor, ensured that his taijiquan would become popular in certain circles. Indeed, some critics believe Zheng style is presently in a weak state because his first generation of students in Taiwan was, on the whole, composed of intellectuals and academics.

Zheng's teaching career in Taiwan spanned a period of twenty-five years, and during this time he taught hundreds, if not thousands, of students. Consequently, students not only reached varying levels of skill but also brought to the art different interests and expectations.

The most obvious differences are in the appearance of the form. Those who learned with him in the earlier years practice a form more closely resembling that of the Yang family, while later students perform in a softer, more rounded fashion. There is much dispute among these students as to whose form is more authentic, although on the whole this tends to be debated rather than contested in more physical terms.

The one exception to this is the case of the dispute between Wu Guozhong and Chen Zichen (a.k.a. William C. C. Chen). Chen started learning from Zheng while still a young boy, even living at his house for a while. Later he went to America, where he developed a large following.

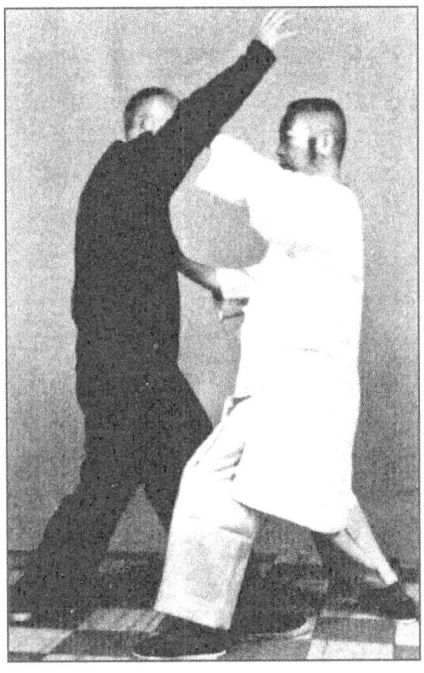

An application of fair lady works at shuttles.

Wu Guozhong, by contrast, only became a disciple fourteen months before Zheng's death, although by his own report he had been training with him for a period of five years or so (Wu: n.d.). Wu claimed, after Zheng's death, to be the only disciple to have learned the "real" taijiquan. Obviously this claim angered many of his fellow disciples, and this was further compounded by the fact that he was extremely successful, collecting thousands of students throughout Southeast Asia. Finally, in the late eighties, matters came to a head and Chen Zichen took up the gauntlet on behalf of his martial art brothers and sought to arrange a match with Wu. After much dispute over the rules, referees, and formalities, nothing was finally agreed, but the whole incident serves as an illustration of the tensions existing in the Zheng system after his death.

There had, however, been tension prior to Zheng's death, one cause being his decision in the midsixties to leave Taiwan for the United States. While the reasons for his move are known among many of his Chinese disciples, they are personal and are not commonly spoken of. Suffice it to say that, to the possible surprise of many of his Western students, it was not for altruistic reasons or to share his art with the world.

Many of his later Chinese students were eager to know just what he taught while in America, and particularly among second- and third-generation students in the East, any information about the nature of his teaching is zealously sought, as are any films featuring him.

No discussion of Zheng's career would be complete without mention of Robert W. Smith, who studied with him in Taiwan and, through his books and articles, made Zheng's taijiquan prowess known through the English-speaking world.

When Zheng's taijiquan was introduced to Malaysia, the pragmatic attitude of the martial arts there necessitated that visiting teachers be prepared to demonstrate the practical applications of their skills. This was because, for historical and political reasons, the Chinese regard themselves as a threatened minority in Malaysia. They are, it is true, in a minority, and certainly there has been oppression, mostly political and occasionally physical, which has provided some justification for their fears. This oppression has resulted in a wholehearted embracing of traditional Chinese culture, whether remembered and passed down from generation to generation or imported by Chinese experts, initially from Taiwan but more recently from mainland China.

The majority of Chinese immigrants arrived during the British colonial rule and hailed from the southern provinces of Fujian and Guangdong. Once in Malaysia they settled primarily in dialect groupings, reproducing the settlement patterns of their native land. Thus, one finds Kuala Lumpur and Ipoh predominantly populated by Cantonese speakers, while in Johor Baru the Chinese are mainly speakers of the Fujian dialect.

The immigrants went to Malaysia fleeing injustice and starvation, or sometimes even as indentured slaves. They were primarily from the lower strata of society and generally in China had little or no access to the so-called higher aspects of their culture (Pan, 1991).[4]

Over the years, however, the descendants of those immigrants have prospered and laid the foundations for the emergence of Malaysia's thriving economy. And with their increasing prosperity they have sought to protect and develop their Chinese identity. This has meant the establishment of private schools; the sponsorship of cultural events, such as Chinese opera, art, and calligraphy exhibitions; the establishment and continued support of religious institutions; and the teaching of Chinese martial arts.

In the case of the latter, there was already a strong foundation in place from the early days of the first mass migrations. The clan wars that raged throughout the southern provinces of China during the nineteenth century resulted in mass migration, both voluntary and involuntary, and these disputes, which pitted village against village and dialect group against dialect group, spilled over into the new land so that age-old feuds were continued on foreign soil (Pan, 1991). Many of the masters I have interviewed in the course of my research have recounted tales of "experts" from China being "imported" to solve problems or train students from a particular dialect group so they might defend themselves against other Chinese!

Master Ng Kionghing, a member of the Hakka dialect group who teaches taijiquan in the southern Malaysian town of Batu Pahat, told me his teacher of Li Jia boxing had been invited over from China by fellow Hakka from his region to help protect them. This same master pursued a vendetta against a master of Hong Jia boxing from a neighboring town, ostensibly over lion dance performance rights, but more probably because several generations earlier a master of the Li style had been beaten by the famed Huang Feihong, the grandmaster of the Hong Jia teacher in the next town.

The settling of disputes through gongfu continues well into the twentieth century, and it was only the increasing prevalence of modern firearms that put traditional fighting skills on the back shelf. The years of fighting and skill testing, however, had established in the Malaysian Chinese martial arts community an attitude of putting one's money where his mouth is and determining the efficacy of technique rather than relying on discussions of philosophy and theory.

While it could be argued that this emphasis on practical application is generally true of Chinese martial arts, the trend, certainly in the latter part of the twentieth century, was to emphasize the healthful and recreational aspects of the arts. Both in Taiwan and China, standardization and an overemphasis on the aesthetics of movement have resulted in a general watering down of the combat elements of the arts.

To a certain extent Zheng himself was involved in this process in Taiwan, but due to his reputation as a person with fighting prowess, a somewhat paradoxical situation arose: while attempting to promote the more cultured aspects of his art, he recruited the majority of his better students by defeating them in challenges of one form or another. Wu Guozhong, Ong Zichuan, and Yue Shuting all reported it was because of losing to Zheng that they became his disciples.

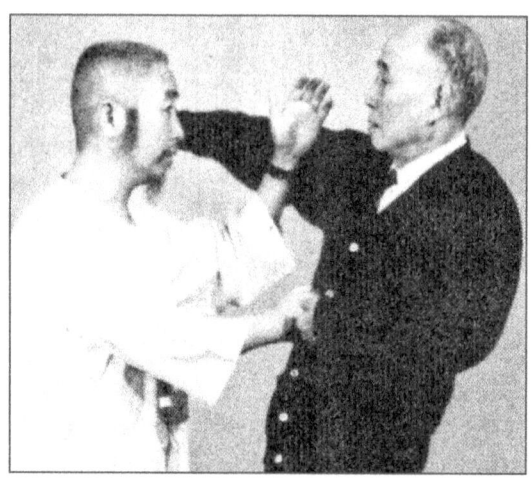

After step forward, deflect downward,
Zheng follows with the parry and punch sequence.

Probably the first teacher to introduce Zheng's taijiquan to what was then Malaya was Huang Xingxian. A native of Fuzhou Province, he had previously studied Fujian White Crane Boxing and in 1955 was taken by one of Zheng's disciples, Yue Shuting, to become a disciple himself. Then in 1956, he went to Singapore and started teaching. A year later Yue Shuting also went to the Malayan peninsula, visiting Penang, where he decided to settle down and start teaching. Yue was originally from Wenzhou in Zhejiang Province, the same area Zheng came from, and prior to meeting Zheng he had studied Shaolin Boxing. He started studying taijiquan with Zheng in the late 1940s in China.

Yue Shuting was responsible for starting a taijiquan dynasty that produced probably the strongest fighters in Malaysia and did much to promote the art as a truly effective fighting style. A small man who photographs reveal as thinner and even shorter than Zheng, himself not very tall, Yue soon made a reputation for himself by taking on and beating all comers.

Li Beilei, a teacher renowned throughout Malaysia for his fighting prowess, trained briefly with Yue Shuting before going on to become a disciple of Yue's most famous disciple, Lu Tongbao. Li recalls it was the fact that he was soundly beaten by this little man that made him give up the Shaolin Luohan boxing he had been practicing and take up taijiquan.[5]

When Yue went to Malaysia, he took with him an old friend from China who had trained in Yang style and who taught the *sanshou* (dispersing hands) two-person form, which Zheng did not teach. Gradually two-person sanshou came to be accepted as a part of Yue's teachings. He also reintroduced some of the moves Zheng himself had omitted, stringing them together into a sequence of eighteen movements he added to the end of the form and simply called the "lower eighteen hands."

These changes reportedly caused Zheng some sadness[6] and he is supposed to have said that some of his students had seen fit to add on extra movements while he, an old man with fifty years of experience, was only really clear about the movements up to the first cross hands (less than a third of the way into the form!). Yue, however, continued to teach his way and, in fact, always referred to what he taught as Yang style. Indeed, some of his students report that when he first started teaching in Penang, it was the traditional Yang long form he taught.[7]

Yue died on June 16, 1975, only a few months after Zheng Manqing. He was in his midsixties and suffering from complications associated with a hole in his heart, which he had from birth. Sadly, he was in Thailand at the time because he had been forced to leave Malaysia due to immigration problems that some aver were deliberately stirred up by jealous rivals.

His most famous student, however, outlived him by another nine years, and was able to pass on Master Yue's unique approach to the art. Lu Tongbao, a heavily built native of Fuqing city, who had previously studied Fujian dog boxing and who owned a tea shop in Penang, trained a whole generation of teachers who are still active throughout Malaysia. Lu died in the early 1980s, but not before he had taught the likes of Li Beilei, Lim Suowei and his brother Lim Souyuan, Chen Huayi, and Lau Kimhong. All of these students suffered and learned at the not-so-gentle hands of Master Lu. Indeed, Lau Kimhong recounts that their sparring mainly consisted of Lu beating them up.[8]

In 1958 Zheng Manqing himself visited Malaysia and Singapore, staying for several months and, according to Song Zijian and Zheng's Malaysian students, teaching a set of neigong exercises that had not previously been taught to his disciples in Taiwan. For some of the time he stayed with Lu Tongbao in Penang, but he also visited Kuala Lumpur, where he gave a demonstration in the Jing Wu stadium, inviting challengers from the audience to come and "try" his gongfu—swiftly and effectively vanquishing all such attempts. After this, Zheng-style taijiquan in Malaysia developed in two main streams: that of Yue Shuting/Lu Tongbao and that of Huang Xingxian.

In the 1980s another teacher appeared on the scene, Wu Guozhong, a former Nationalist soldier who claimed to have learned the "real" Zheng-style taijiquan. His high tuition was based on this claim. Teaching his disciples what he claimed to be the authentic teachings of Zuo Laipeng, he charged anything between $1,000 and $2,000 of the local currency to people wishing to become his disciples, after which they would become eligible to learn the "secrets." The bad blood caused by his claims and by his material success culminated in the previously mentioned challenge match with Chen Zichen. In the meantime, exponents from the Yue/Lu stream had not been idle. Taking exception to his statement in a Malaysian national Chinese-language newspaper that Malaysian taijiquan had gone down a blind alley and was nothing more than dancing, Li Beilei, Zhou Mutu, and Lim Souyuan went to "call" on him during a talk he was giving. They invited Wu to prove his ability with actions instead of words. Unable, for whatever reason, to meet their challenge, in the pragmatic climate of the Malaysian Chinese martial arts world, Wu quietly faded from the scene. Of the several thousands who had flocked to become his disciples, most were disappointed by his failure to prove himself and to reveal any "secrets" of real value, and only two or three hundred are now left.

Each of the three main streams has its unique characteristics. Practitioners from the Yue Shuting tradition tend to emphasize more "muscular" taijiquan and are active on the tournament scene. In both of the last two international taijiquan championships held in Taiwan, the Malaysian team has been almost exclusively made of exponents of this tradition. Their attitude seems to be very much one of taking what works and applying it, whether it be to push-hands or fighting.

The Huang Xingxian stream in Malaysia, prompted in recent years by Huang's own demonstrations of his seeming ability to send his students flying with just a twitch of his finger, has degenerated into a limp parody of the skill that Huang was reputed to have had in his earlier days. However, in Taiwan, exponents of Huang's approach to taijiquan demonstrate a much more realistic approach to the art with a proven ability in both push-hands and application. The situation that has arisen and perpetuated among Huang's students in Malaysia is due to one of those cases of apparent mass hypnosis that occur periodically in the world of martial arts, whereby a first generation of adoring and overawed students place all their faith in a master figure and attribute their initial lack of expertise and inevitable defeat at the hands of the master to some almost magical power they feel the master will always have over them. This belief then becomes fixed so that, almost despite their best efforts, they feel unable to gain the master's skill. Indeed, the students come to feel this would be impossible because the master has the "power."

This situation then becomes institutionalized, with each successive generation of students "teaching" their successors to respond to the master's touch in the appropriate way. Thus, in many videotapes one can view Huang merely tapping his students, who then engage in gymnastic contortions as they hurl themselves across the room with looks of awe and wonder on their faces. Sadly, in his later years Huang, who died in 1992, seems to have believed in his own ability to perform these amazing feats. When he occasionally encountered those who would not throw themselves at his slightest touch, he either sought to intimidate them by striking them as he pushed with them, or to attribute their failure to "fly" to a high level of gongfu on their part.[9]

Wu Guozhong's students have, however, gone one step further, falling back on a hoary old chestnut: "We cannot practice freestyle push-hands with people outside our school because our qi might damage them." Their reliance on such arguments suggests that the role of hard physical work (gongfu) has been all but eliminated from their training program. Inspired perhaps by their master's stories of the secrets of the "real" Zheng style that he alone learned, at present they rely mainly on long-winded and intellectual expositions of just what exactly their taijiquan is all about, rather than developing the solid skills that would substantiate their claims.

The three main streams of Zheng style may be further characterized according to the different emphasis of each group. Because of the rough and ready atmosphere that existed at the time Yue Shuting started teaching, a tradition was swiftly established in which exponents proved the validity of their art in a practical and sometimes violent manner. While students of this stream, particularly those who learned from Lu Tongbao, still adhere to this philosophy, there has been a tendency among some students on the periphery of this group to become uneasy about the inability of their teachers to explain the finer points of the theory and philosophy that are the foundation of the art. Thus, these students have often found themselves in a seemingly never-ending search for a teacher who can both explain the principles and apply them. This search has led many to mainland China, yet few have found the satisfaction they seek, as the world of taijiquan is littered with fine "talkers" who prove to be less than adequate "doers."[10]

While Huang started teaching in Malaysia at the same time as Yue, whether by accident or design, he ended up with a different type of student, many of whom seemed to be in search of magic and were not too curious about the exact nature of this magic. A number of sources I have interviewed in the course of my research have pointed out that, while the successors of Yue Shuting have gone on to carve out reputations for themselves as master instructors in their own right, none of Huang's students has done the same. Indeed, among his students there is very much a cult of the master.[11]

Wu Guozhong, coming later to the scene with his promise of access to the innermost secrets of Zheng's system, initially attracted students from a wide range of backgrounds, but as his power base in Malaysia became more established, he began to surround himself with intellectuals and high-level businessmen. Cynically, one could observe that these people not only offered the most in terms of material advantage but also posed the least physical threat. Indeed, many of his current students are particularly attracted by the intellectual and highbrow approach he takes in his teaching. Currently one of Wu's leading students, Dr. Wong Bingfeng, teaches a course in taijiquan and related Chinese philosophy at the Malaysian Institute of Arts, a private tertiary education institute in Kuala Lumpur.

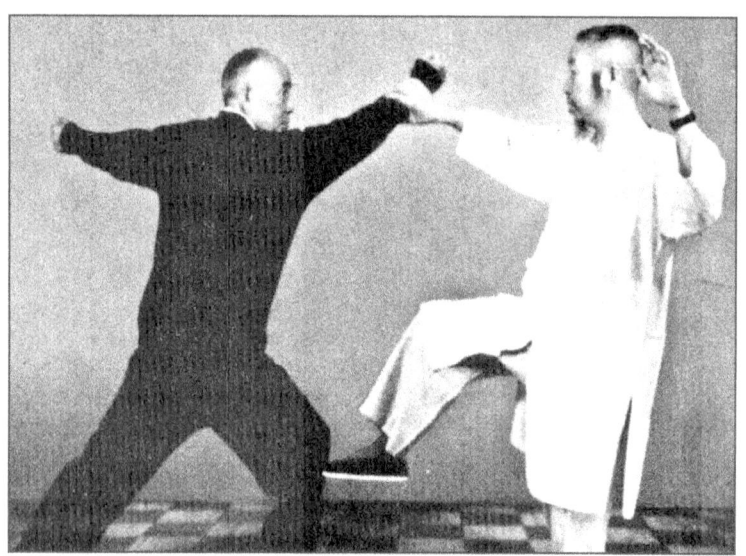

An application of separate right foot.

In the last two years, Wu's organization has been further weakened by the departure of his chief instructor, Koh Ahtee. Koh might well be typical of the new generation of adherents to the Zheng style, as his training career has constantly centered on the desire to learn as much as possible about what Zheng actually taught. Koh's defection, taking with him many of Wu's senior students, decimated Wu's Shenlong Association.

Koh Ahtee is interesting to anyone wanting to speculate about the future of Zheng style in Malaysia, as he has trained extensively in both Wu Guozhong and Lu Tongbao streams. He started studying taijiquan at the age of fourteen, becoming a disciple of Master Lau Kimhong, who was himself a disciple of Lu Tongbao. Lau, intent on proving the efficacy of taijiquan, had early in his career entered a Southeast Asian full-contact fighting championship and taken second in his category, only failing to get first place because of disqualification.

The young Koh impressed Master Lau with his hard-working attitude, and soon he had become one of his best students. Accompanying Lau Kimhong on trips to his various classes around southern Malaysia, Koh had plenty of opportunities to learn from the best of Master Lau's contemporaries. Then, hearing about Wu Guozhong's claims, Koh Ahtee sought him out. At that time, however, Wu was not in Singapore, but Master Tan Chingngee was taking disciples on his behalf. In the Zheng tradition as promulgated by Wu, disciples were often taken into the tradition but not directly by the teacher concerned. Master Tan had visited Taiwan when only eighteen years old in 1974. While there he had trained with Zheng and, according to some, had become his disciple. This claim is open to dispute, but Koh to this day believes it to be true. Wanting to learn more of what Zheng actually taught, Koh asked Master Tan if he could become his disciple. This was highly irregular, as Koh was already a disciple of Master Lau and, furthermore, Master Lau and Master Tan had been friends for a number of years.

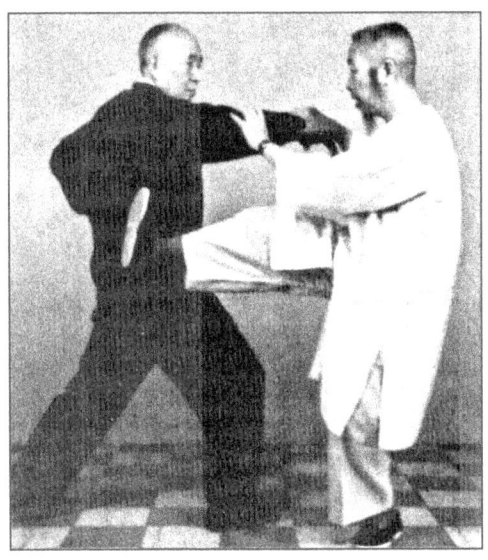

An application of turn body and sweep lotus with leg.

Out of respect for Master Lau, Koh told him of his intention to become a disciple and Master Lau, furious at his student, punished him by making him kneel in front of a picture of Zhang Sanfeng for several hours. Then, when Wu reappeared on the Malaysian scene after working in America, Koh announced to Master Tan his intention of becoming Wu's disciple. Now it was Master Tan's turn to be furious with his promising student, but all to no avail, for Koh had made up his mind. Showing the same dedication to training that he had with his previous teachers, he swiftly rose to become chief instructor for Wu's Shenlong Association in Kuala Lumpur.

Finally, disillusioned with what he saw as the widening gap between the teachings of Wu and the original doctrine of Zheng Manqing, Koh left to set up as an independent instructor in his own right. Since then he has sought to adhere strictly to Zheng's teachings and has become a successful professional instructor. Being only in his midthirties, he may be able to reach the highest levels of the art. Indeed, Koh might prove to be the helmsman for a new generation, a new breed of Zheng stylist, combining as he does the "show me" attitude of the Yue Shuting stream with the purism and strong theoretical and philosophical base of the Wu Guozhong stream.

Utterly unintimidated by other martial artists of any discipline, Koh is always willing to demonstrate his skills in whatever fashion is the most appropriate, and in his constant search for more knowledge, he seeks out practitioners of taijiquan with a reputation for having gongfu and seeks to determine whether the reputation is deserved.

Prior to the 1990s, Zheng style was probably the most popular style of taijiquan in Malaysia, due not only to the efforts of the three streams described above, but also to the relative underexposure to other styles caused by the political situation in Malaysia. In response to the years of the Emergency, when war was waged against the communist guerrillas, the Chinese population came under suspicion and the Chinese government's support of the rebels meant not only did Malaysia have no diplomatic ties with the country, but her Chinese citizens were not allowed to visit the motherland until after retirement. It was only after the final surrender of the remaining communists at the end of the 1980s that this ruling was relaxed and Chinese of all ages could visit China. This political change also opened the doors to a flood of martial arts coaches from the People's Republic of China who previously had only been permitted to teach in Singapore. The new market proved particularly profitable for them, and they now visit in a constant stream, so representatives of all the major styles may now be found running variously thriving associations throughout Malaysia.

Since the mid-1980s there have also been an increasing number of competitions held in Malaysia. These range from competitions only for taijiquan forms and push-hands using Taiwan rules, to the mainland Chinese–inspired *wushu* competitions, with their standardized forms and emphasis on aesthetics. The presence of these competitions has further divided Zheng stylists with, as might be expected, the Yue Shuting/Lu Tongbao descendants entering and enjoying considerable success, while both Wu's students and Huang's have, on the whole, been critical and reluctant to participate.

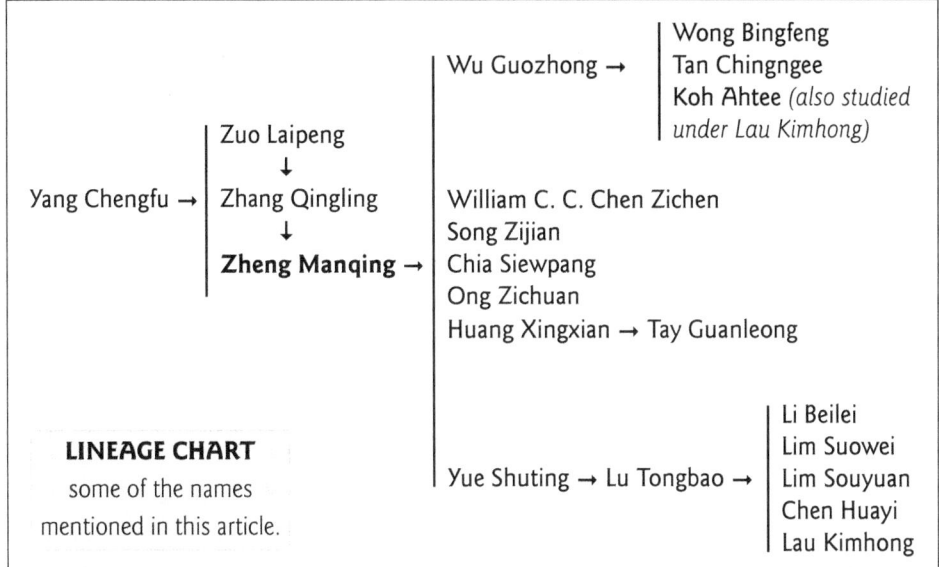

LINEAGE CHART
some of the names mentioned in this article.

What then are the major differences in training methodology among the groups? As has already been mentioned, practitioners of the Yue stream refer to their art as Yang style, although most of them have given up teaching the long form. Zhou Mutu reported to me that this is due to the lack of patience of present-day students.[12] They do, however, teach broadsword, which was not a part of Zheng's curriculum. Straight sword is also taught, but not staff or spear. The sanshou solo and two-person forms are taught after the taijiquan solo form and the lower eighteen hands have been learned. Push-hands features prominently with both a series of basic exercises and freestyle being taught. Although the *peng-lu-ji-an* (ward-off, rollback, press, push) pattern that was such a vital part of Zheng's curriculum is known, it is not emphasized.

The disciple system is still used widely, although some teachers, such as Li Beilei, have simplified the ceremony while retaining the essence, namely that there is a body of knowledge that is not openly taught. At the heart of this "secret knowledge" is the system of qigong and body conditioning taught by Zheng to Lu Tongbao during his trip to Malaysia in 1958. Many outsiders and even Zheng stylists from Taiwan have denied that such a system existed and say it comes from "external style" martial arts and was probably introduced by Lu himself. Whether this is true or not, all of the exponents I have interviewed hold strongly to the view that it came from Zheng. Having talked to people from the different branches of Zheng style as well as those in Taiwan, I have concluded there are enough similarities in methodology to suggest the system did in fact come from Zheng; such similarities include emphasis on relaxation and gradual progress.

In schools of the Yue/Lu stream, the art is still emphasized as martial in origin and application, and it is not unusual to find sandbags hung in the training hall and on occasion some form of sparring included in the training for senior students. No great emphasis is placed on philosophical explanations or detailed examination of theory; instead the emphasis is very much on the practical. Perhaps because of this, the students tend to be younger than in other schools, the average age being between twenty-eight and thirty-eight.

In Huang's schools a great deal of time is spent on achieving the elusive state of song (relaxation), with a number of auxiliary exercises created by Huang prominent in the curriculum. Practitioners of this stream practice their form at a slower pace than most other exponents, arguing that this better enables them to concentrate on song. Huang also devised his own fast form for practicing applications, but how widely this is taught I do not know, only that some exponents make reference to it.

Huang was reputedly very traditional and secretive, and he certainly took disciples. Indeed, one of his senior students, Master Tay Guanleong, told me when he first approached Huang about becoming a student, after thinking it over, Huang invited him to come and live in his house for three months so he could observe him firsthand and decide whether he were worthy.[13] Other members on the periphery of Huang's organization seem less certain about the value of such secrecy, advocating the open sharing of knowledge and, where their understanding is limited, borrowing from a wide range of sources.[14]

While weapons such as the straight sword are taught, undoubtedly the most important aspects of Huang's approach to Zheng style are the solo form and auxiliary qigong. Push-hands exercises and freestyle push-hands are both taught, but many of Huang's students, instead of spending their time building a solid foundation, seek to reproduce Huang's magical feats and suffer some discouragement when failing to do so.

The curriculum taught to students in the Wu stream follows what Wu claims to have learned from Zheng, consisting of form, push-hands, and straight sword. A system of qigong is also taught using sandalwood for massage of vital points. As mentioned before, the training emphasizes theory and philosophy, and there is not much room for physical experimentation.

The whole question of application is treated in an abstract manner, an approach that is justified according to Zheng's own writings. In a section on sanshou in the *Thirteen Chapters*, he wrote: "If one is able to interpret energy and master the techniques, one's applications will be successful" (Lo & Inn: 1985). What he does not reveal, however, is exactly how to "interpret energy and master the techniques."

At present, Zheng style in Malaysia is going through further changes. The death of Huang Xingxian has precipitated a power struggle among his students, despite the fact that, prior to his death, he named his son-in-law as his successor. Wu Guozhong still visits Malaysia from time to time, but his arrival is no longer heralded by large-scale publicity, as it once was. The majority of Lu Tongbao's students who are now teaching are in their fifties and seem to be enjoying some success in training a new generation of students. Their competitive spirit now serves as a major focus for both the development and recognition of skill.

Whatever happens in the future, however, the unique circumstances of the Malaysian Chinese—their desire to explore their Chinese heritage together with their geographical distance from Taiwan, where Zheng style is arguably stagnant—combine to ensure that Zheng style will continue to grow, evolve, and flourish.

Notes

1. Published in *Full Circle*, a publication compiled by a group of Zheng's former students in the United States after his death. The biography was translated by Tam Gibbs, and the full text in Chinese may be found on the wall of Zheng's tomb in Taibei, Taiwan.
2. Personal interview conducted by the author, September 1992, in Taibei, Taiwan.
3. Personal interview conducted by the author, September 1992, in Taibei, Taiwan.
4. For more information on Chinese immigration to Malaysia, see Pan, *Sons of the Yellow Emperor*.
5. Personal interview conducted by the author, June 1991, in Malaysia.
6. Personal interview with Koh Ahtee conducted by the author, February 1993, in Malaysia. Koh as a disciple of Wu Guozhong was told this anecdote by Wu.
7. Personal interview with Li Beilai conducted by the author, June 1991, in Malaysia.
8. Personal interview with Lau Kimhong, June 1991, in Malaysia.
9. Personal interview with Koh Ahtee conducted by the author, February 1993, in Malaysia. Koh had such an experience pushing hands with Huang.
10. In March 1993 a guest teacher from China, teaching a variety of forms of taijiquan and qigong and explaining them in relation to the *Yijing*, found his classes undersubscribed, despite initial enthusiasm, after he was bested in push-hands by a number of local exponents whose skills might best be described, even by themselves, as average.
11. Personal correspondence with a number of his students has confirmed this, as have the squabbles over leadership of his organization that have occurred since

his death, as none of the senior students is perceived as having the same high level of skill.

[12] Personal interview with Zhou Mutu, June 1991, in Malaysia.
[13] Conversation with Tay Guanleong, April 1993.
[14] Private correspondence with Huang's students.

Bibliography

Chia, S., & Goh, E. (1983). *Tai Chi: Ten minutes to health*. Singapore: Times Books International.

Lo, P., & Inn, M. (Trans.). (1985). *Cheng Tzu's thirteen treatises on t'ai chi ch'uan*. New York: North Atlantic Books.

Pan, L. (1991). *The sons of the Yellow Emperor: The story of the overseas Chinese*. London: Mandarin.

Wile, D. (Comp. & Trans.). (1985). *Cheng Man-ch'ing's advanced form instructions*. Brooklyn, New York: Sweet Ch'i Press.

Wu, K. (n.d.). *Tao tai chi health*. Self-published.

Zheng Manqing and Taijiquan:
A Clarification of Role
by Robert W. Smith, M.A.

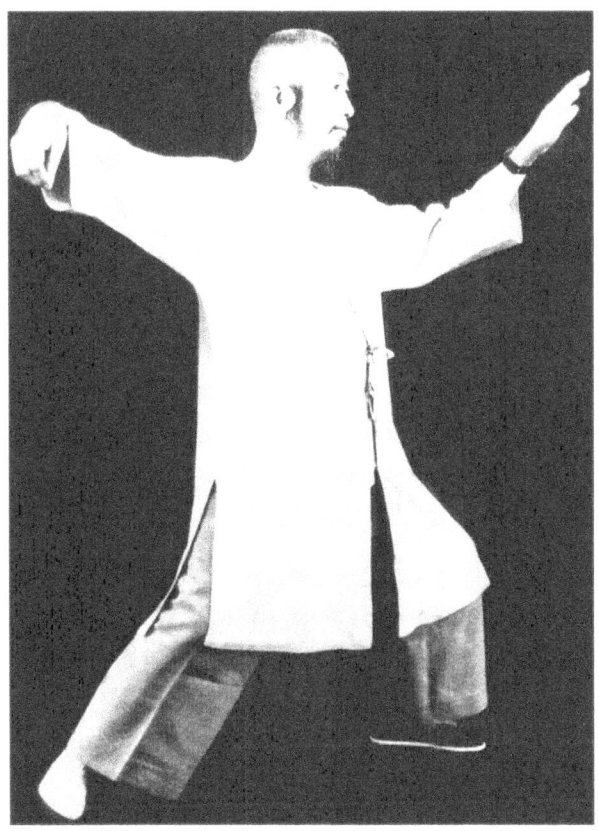

Zheng in single-whip posture, 1965. All illustrations courtesy of R. Smith, and Charles E. Tuttle Co., except where noted.

In his article on Zheng Manqing's taijiquan (hereafter, simply "taiji") in Malaysia, Nigel Sutton makes some errors of fact and interpretation that I would like to correct (1994: 57–71). A guiding principle to help correct Sutton's commentary is that "the teacher is not the taught." The fact that taiji students do a movement in a certain way does not mean that the teacher did it that way or would even agree to it being done that way. Or, by extension, merely because teachers in Malaysia, Taiwan, or America make comments regarding taiji, what they say does not necessarily reflect what Professor Zheng said or would say on a given aspect of the art.

Sutton goes awry in the first paragraph by stating that Zheng Manqing founded a new system of taiji (1994: 57).[1] This is an error. The long form he learned and taught before World War II was exactly that of Yang Chengfu. There is evidence that Zheng may have been experimenting with a shorter form as early as 1938 when he was director of martial arts in Hunan Province. Given wartime exigencies, he shortened the set by eliminating many repetitions and some postures. But it was somewhat later, in 1947, just before he went to Taiwan, that the shorter form came to fruition.

When I was studying with him in Taiwan (1959–1962), I queried him on the genesis and development of his short form. He was convinced that he'd been right to simplify it. That was said smiling. But then he'd get sterner, saying that it was not a creation of a new system, but rather a rearrangement not affecting basic principles. This form, he said, is the shorter Yang Chengfu system taught by one with half his teacher's skill. Sutton views this as a "new system," but Zheng would not call it so.

Sutton next states that it is generally recognized by students of Zheng Manqing that his incorporation of core elements of the Zuo Laipeng system made his system unique (1994: 58). I know of no one who believes this. We know little of Zuo, but we do know that he did not teach taiji.

To understand Zuo, one must first understand another remarkable person: Zhang Qinlin. The best way to learn about both these men, it seems to me, is through Wang Yannian, a taiji teacher I discussed in *Chinese Boxing: Masters and Methods* (1974). In his book *Taichi* (1988, Taibei), Wang tells how, through a Daoist friend, he met Zhang Qinlin, a taiji teacher over sixty at the time, who had jet-black hair and looked forty. Zhang was born in Hebei in 1887 of a poor family and at fourteen became a yardman at the family home of Yang Jianhou. Over the years, the youngster practiced with Yang Chengfu and other adepts there, becoming quite proficient (Wang, 1988: 1–2, 41–42).

In 1914, Wan Laisheng, a senior student of the famed Du Xinwu, traveled through Hunan and, when he came to Hubei, challenged Yang Chengfu. Zhang took the challenge for Yang and defeated Wan in the first clash—probably injuring Wan's arm.[2] Wan decamped.

Yang Jianhou, who watched the skirmish from inside his house, was taken by Zhang's bravery and skill in beating Wan. Wang Yannian believes that Yang Jianhou's appreciation was also stimulated by the fact that years before Yang himself had a match with Du Xinwu, Wan's teacher, which ended in a stalemate. Lacking corroboration, I tend to doubt that such a match ever occurred.

Be that as it may, Wang writes that Jianhou demonstrated his appreciation by secretly showing Zhang the original Han style of taiji that his father, Yang

Luchan, had concealed from the Manchu court when he taught there. Luchan had taught an inferior method, keeping the original Han style for family use only.

Later, Zhang Qinlin met Zuo Laipeng of the Golden Elixir of Life School who taught him neigong (internal work) and *tunu daoyin* (breathing methods) esoteric skills.[3] These Zhang blended with his taiji abilities and his skill became great. In *Chinese Boxing* I tell how Zhang traveled, defeating all boxers until he met Zuo, who tumbled him instantly, commenting, "Your technique, sir, is none too good."[4] Although Wang does not mention the encounter, it is widely believed.

Zhang went to Taiyuan in Shanxi in 1925 to work as a fur merchant and prospered. In the 1929 national martial arts championships held at Nanjing, Zhang, the Shanxi Province champion, became the national champion as well. It is said that he won the honor without breaking a sweat and afterwards berated the principals for not affording him stiffer competition.

Wang Yannian visited me in 1984 and I was able to ask him about Zhang's relationship with Zheng Manqing. After the Nanjing tournament, Wang said, Professor Zheng approached Zhang Qinlin and asked to study under him. Zhang told Zheng that, since he was already versed in taiji, he would accept him as a student and let him live at his house in Taiyuan but without the customary kowtow.[5]

Wang told me that, physically, Zhang Qinlin was midway between Zheng Manqing and Wang himself but that he had big wide feet, huge hands that seemed to cover one's chest, and was a supple as a snake. His description of Zhang's feet rang a bell: I had heard in Taiwan that he could root so well that his feet actually sank into the ground. This was the colossus who taught Zheng push-hands and qigong for six months. At the end of the period, Zheng imprudently suggested that they have a real go and was soundly drubbed by Zhang.

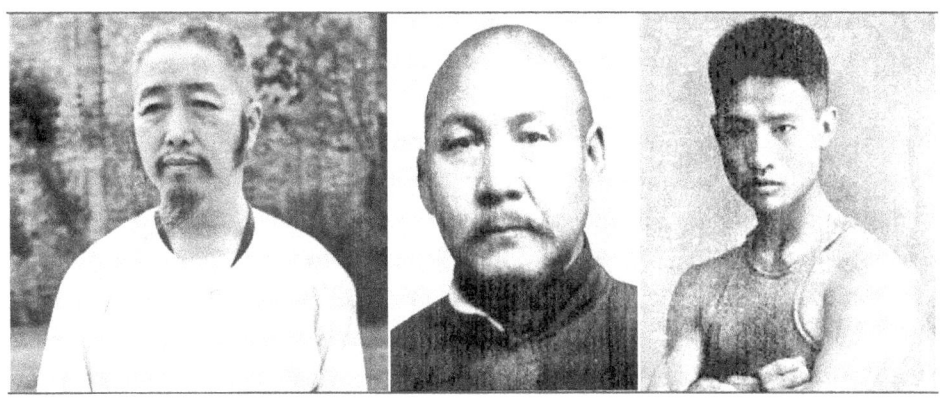

Left: Professor Zheng in 1960. Center: Zhang Qinlin—who taught Zheng neigong (photo courtesy of Wang Yannian). Right: Wan Laisheng.

Some of Zheng's senior students, however, view Zhang Qinlin differently than Wang Yannian did. Liu Xiheng and Ben Lo (Pangjeng) believe that Zheng primarily studied neigong, rather than push-hands, from Zhang and that it was done in Shanghai rather than Shanxi. They reason that, though Zheng practiced push-hands with Zhang as students under Yang Chengfu, his main priority was learning neigong, probably including Zuo Laipeng's teaching, from Zhang.[6] The place may not be important, but it is worth noting that the memorial book of Zheng states that in Taiyuan, Shanxi, he "practiced marvelous techniques of [taiji] energy with [Zhang Qinlin]" (Gibbs, 1985: 18).[7] Mrs. Zheng, however, says that Professor Zheng did not study in Shanxi. Coming from such a strong source, this statement, besides negating Wang Yannian's assertion, adds some weight to the general belief that Zheng never actually met Zuo Laipeng but, instead, derived his neigong from Zhang Qinlin outside of Shanxi, where both Zhang and Zuo lived.

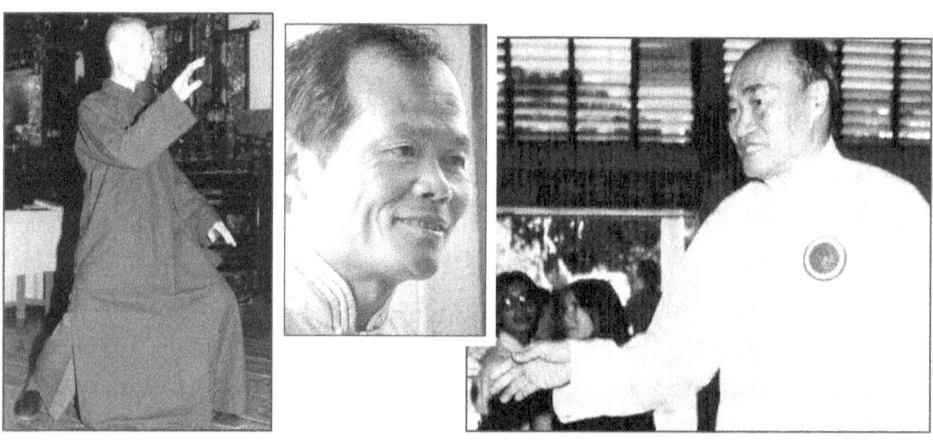

Left: Liu Xiheng—student and confidant of Zheng. Center: Ben Lo.
Right: Huang Xingxian—Zheng's student who spread taiji in Malaysia.

Moreover, Liu Xiheng and Ben Lo say that, when Zhang Qinlin came to Yang Chengfu, he had already learned another taiji form. Yang accepted him and told him that because his form was so good (Professor Zheng told Mr. Liu Xiheng once that it was "very soft, very beautiful") that he needn't study form but only push-hands. Liu further writes, "Some people say this is a secret Yang Family form, but Master Yang's son has denied this and has indicated that it is only Mr. [Zhang's] form." As for Zheng Manqing's challenge to Zhang, as related by Wang Yannian, Liu says, "Perhaps not too much should be made of it, as it would be in the natural order of things in the push-hands class, where these things shift back and forth from day to day."[8]

But what of the mystery man Zuo Laipeng? In his book *Writings on the Way of Taichi*, Wu Guozhong wrote that Zheng Manqing created a new system from a synthesis of Zuo style, Yang style, and his own unique system. This is a major mistake made, one hopes, from carelessness rather than self-serving commercialism. Ben Lo's article in *T'ai Chi* magazine (Lo, 1985) criticizes Wu Guozhong for promoting this error. In his polite but devastating analysis, Lo quotes these words from Professor Zheng's seminal *Thirteen Treatises on Taichi* (Lo, 1985):

> This book is the result of my teacher Professor Yang Chengfu and his taichi book, *T'i Yung Ch'uan Shu*. This book follows my teacher's instructions and is a continuation of his book. Because the traditional form was too long, people lacking patience could not easily finish it and did not continue practicing. Therefore, I simplified the form by deleting the repetitions which were about 70 percent of the form. I called my work *Simplified Taichi*. My classmate, Ch'en Weiming, encouraged my book and urged me to publish it. I believe this work is in harmony with my teacher's idea.

How could Wu, who must have read the *Thirteen Treatises*, miss this passage? Lo then cites Wu Guozhong's book, which quotes a crucial sentence from Zheng Manqing's *Manjan San Lun* written in 1971:

> My fellow student Ch'en Hsiao-lien [Weiming] studied T'ai chi ch'uan for several decades, but when it came to the difference between strength and energy, he was not able to get to the bottom of it. Not long after that I received the secret teaching of Master [Zuo Laipeng of Shanxi] which stated that the strength issues from the bones, but energy issues from the sinews. In a burst of clarity I was enlightened. Forty years ago I wrote these words in my *Master Cheng's Thirteen Chapters on Tai-chi ch'üan* . . .
> —Wile, 1985: 148

In fact, Professor Zheng cites the same quote twice in this book (Lo & Inn, 1985: 79, 91). In neither case is it claimed that the words came from Zuo Laipeng. Lo suggests that Professor Zheng may have actually gotten the words he attributes to Zuo from Zhang Qinlin, student of Zuo's neigong and Yang's push-hands method.

Lo writes that the quote is probably a part of the Yang family tradition rather than the esoteric Daoist one. As proof, he cites Wu Gongzao's *Wu Style Taichi* (1980), which included a photo reproduction of a written manuscript "On Methods of Taichi" passed along by the author's ancestor, Wu Jianquan, who had received it from Yang Banhou. All told, it had been in the Wu family for more than one hundred years (Lo, "Explanation," 1985: 12).⁹ The same document was included by Dong Yingjie, a senior student of Yang Chengfu, in his *Taichi Shih-i* [Explanation of tai chi] (1948), thirty-two years earlier.

To Wu Guozhong's contention that he had "learned a final, concentration distillation of fifty years of Professor [Zheng's] experience," Ben Lo answers that there was no difference between the postures of earlier and later periods. "There is only the difference between postures correctly learned and incorrectly learned." Then Lo concludes that Wu "remains inadequate in even the most superficial aspects of the art" (Lo, 1985: 17).

Later, Wu had the temerity to challenge aging Huang Xingxian of Singapore, but this fight was not consummated. (As the challenged given the choice of weapons, Huang should have accepted and specified push-hands in which—even factoring in age—he was clearly superior to Wu.) In due course, Wu's perceived misdeeds brought a challenge from William Chen. After a long play in Chinese newspapers, the pair was unable to agree on modalities and this challenge also fizzled.

The episode hurt everyone and did not help Professor Zheng's reputation. I have always held the view that the Wu-Chen disagreement could likewise have been solved by push-hands (*tuishou*). Since push-hands confirms one's form, a round of it would settle most points in the controversy. A tuishou match is still a possibility. (I suggested this recently to a student of Wu and got this response: "A spot of tuishou? Well, in the last couple months, Wu has published in Chinese in Taiwan a two-hundred-plus-page book on push-hands, which is selling fast. One of the things about this guy is that he doesn't keep secrets." What does a book tell about one's abilities?) If Wu is as bad at taiji as some suggest, then it will be known soon enough. But, if that is true, then Wu already knows and will steer clear of the sportive and opt for what his followers think is his strong suit—the free fight. According to Sutton, Wu's reputation is that of a Chinese military frogman "who has killed many men" (1994: 64). So why wouldn't he respond to a challenge brought by three of Lu Tongbao's students? The whole affair is full of confusion. I have heard that Wu has recanted the claims attributed to him that stated he was the sole inheritor of Zheng's most important teachings. The evidence adduced against him by Lo and others is far too weighty to perpetuate such claims.¹⁰

Sutton also writes that Professor Zheng's thirty-seven postures "are based closely, if only superficially, on the Yang style" (1994: 58). This sentence is a paradox and contradicts what Zheng has stated regarding the influence of Yang Chengfu.

Lower on the same page, Sutton claims that the Zuo system places a greater emphasis on song (relaxation) than does the Yang style. We know that a Zuo system of taiji does not exist, but we do not know with any clarity what Zuo's neigong method involved. We do know, however, that the Yang system puts a premium on relaxation.

The Yang system regarded the *Taichi Classics* as its bible, which contains such statements as Wu Yuxiang's "The softest will then become the strongest" (Lo, et al., 1979: 46). Reflecting Yang Chengfu's direct teaching, Chen Weiming says in *Questions and Answers on Taichi*, "Students who use force can't believe that at the limit of suppleness lies a different quality of strength," and, "A poor student is hard and uses force but a good one must be supple without force" (Lo & Smith, 1985: 18). Finally, Professor Zheng says in his *Thirteen Treatises* that Yang Chengfu repeated continually, "Relax! Relax! Relax completely" (Lo & Inn, 1985: 88). I know Sutton joins me in wishing we could relax better. He is right, I think, in believing that Zuo's neigong helped Professor Zheng's taiji. In fact, Zheng acknowledged as much. But we just do not know how or to what degree these practices intertwined.

Given its Daoist beginnings, we should not be surprised at change in taiji as it evolves and proliferates. Even in the short form, no two teachers do the form exactly alike. Sutton, like some other recent writers, thinks he sees a difference between earlier and later Zheng style: "Those who learned with him in the earlier years practice a form more closely resembling that of the Yang family while later students perform [sic] in a softer, more rounded fashion" (1994: 22). This, he says, led some exponents of the Yang system to accuse Zheng stylists of, doing "old man's taiji." However, Zheng taught as Yang had taught him. Both had students of varied ages and varied taiji skills.

One must distinguish the teacher from the taught. Sutton thinks Zheng Manqing softened and rounded the Yang postures, but Yang was far softer then Zheng. And the fact that some of Zheng's students do postures one way does not mean Zheng taught them that way. Isn't it just possible that Zheng's teachings involved no changes, but instead simply reflects that he was superb at not changing Yang's system, teaching it as he had learned it? Zheng stressed accuracy first and last. When he learned the rudiments under Yang, he had to master each posture before moving to the next; there was no breezy form class followed by a corrections class. With time, his own form became less energetic and more internalized—compare his 1960 Taiwan film with his 1973 film—but his teaching remained pretty much the same.

I learned and taught taiji across thirty-five years with Professor Zheng and his influence early and late, and must correct Sutton on misstatements regarding form. Above all, this must be stressed: the Zheng form is the Yang form shortened, but the postures—the structure and flow—and the principles are all the same.

Without being didactic, let me dilate on the form. Everyone's form will be different—like fingerprints or snowflakes—but the basics will be the same. The structure will be pretty much the same while the flow will come to express some of the personality of the person doing it. Together these two elements comprise the technique of taiji. Professor Zheng would ask taiji practitioners: how much of taiji technique is structure and how much is flow. The answer is that early in one's training, as one learns to apply the basics, structure predominates, but later, flow comes to the fore. Professor Zheng would go on to say that structure and flow together—the technique—make up only 30 percent of taiji. He would then ask, "What is the missing 70 percent?" It is the same as in many arts, in calligraphy—the queen of the Chinese fine arts—for instance. Seventy percent of taiji is naturalness, the intrinsic "you," which can only come from inside you.

That said, it is obvious that there is a complex of factors operating in taiji. Only some of these are visible to the beginning eye. "It is not that fast horses are rare," said Tang scholar Han Yu. "It's just that those who can really spot them are few."

Now, the art would be difficult—Professor Zheng said that taiji was the most difficult of all his "excellences"—even if there were one standard, undeviating model. But there is not. There are two orthodox streams connecting us with founder Yang Luchan, those of sons Jianhou and Banhou. These systems vary somewhat but are still Yang. Zheng Manqing learned from Yang Chengfu, son of Jianhou. Yang Chengfu had a small cadre of top seniors, ranging from Chen Weiming and Dong Yingjie, the most senior, to Zheng Manqing, the youngest. Each had his own style, but each did the Yang system.

Given the history of the Yang family, one should expect some difference in the system as the result of differences in locale, social milieu, teacher, and other variables. With the underdeveloped agrarian economy and poor communications of China, there were few books on taiji that would have helped standardize the system. And then there were the students. To enhance ego, many would stop learning too early before they really understood taiji well enough to teach it; others would learn a different system and then attach the Yang name to it for prestige; and still others would learn the Yang, change it, and then tag their name to the mongrel system. These aberrations tended to dilute the system in many areas. Both Banhou and Jianhou taught a system that could accommodate all physiques and psyches. The system embraced a big method with a high stance, the arms moving in proportionally larger circles; a medium method having a middle stance with greater separation of weight between the feet, the arms moving in smaller circles; and a small method with the knees deeply bent and the arms moving minimally, most movement being at the waist. Yang Shaohou was proficient in the difficult small method and his trigger-force short energy made him a terror in push-hands. His form was nearly as frightening. A few years ago, a Beijing newspaper interviewed Wu Tunan, a taiji veteran nearing one hundred, who told the interviewer that, when he studied under Yang Shaohou, he was made to do the form under a table for lengthy periods.

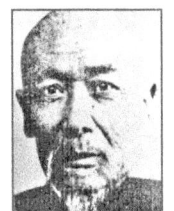 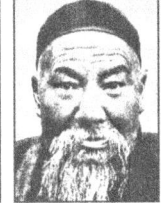 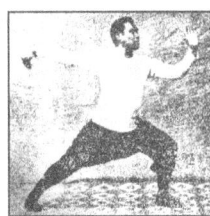

Yang Shaohou, Yang Jianhou (Zheng's grand teacher), and Yang Chengfu, c. 1932.

The key factor distinguishing the low form was simply the height of the form—that is, how much the knees were bent in separating the weight in the stance. I assume, therefore, that the hand position sequence remained essentially the same as in the other forms. I saw a little of this low form in the parks in Taiwan—the hand sequence was the same—but though the players were quite low, the quality of their practice was not too high. Confucius said, germanely, "Some seek Happiness higher than man; others seek it lower. But Happiness is the same height as man."

Continuing our discussion of the form, as time passes, sincere, thinking students will make changes, often contributing beneficially rather than detrimentally to a system's evolution. Something like this occurred in 1938 when Zheng Manqing decided to do as Thoreau advises all of us to, to "simplify, simplify." For largely practical reasons, he reduced the number of postures in a routine from more than a hundred to thirty-seven—still nearly triple the number of postures in the original taiji set (thirteen). And this kind of change is seen in the broad sweep of taiji history.

Chenjiagou, Henan, was the hub of early taiji in China, learning the art from a Shanxi boxer, Wang Zongyue, who visited Henan in the last half of the eigh- teenth century. Much later, taiji at Chenjiagou split into the so-called old (orthodox) and new (innovative) camps. The split was not decisive in its effect on style, however. The principles and postures of the "new" were not dissimilar from those of the "old." Perhaps a more important change occurred at about the same time. Wu Yuxiang, who had learned the "old" taiji from Yang Luchan and the "new" system from Chen Qingping, synthesized these into his own system. What I want to stress here is the active evolution of the "new" system (see chart on pages 202–203 showing the "new" and "old" lineages in Draeger & Smith, 1980). Wu Yuxiang passed his system to Li Yiyu, who passed it to Hao Weizhen, who passed it to Sun Lutang. Each of these masters modified it and renamed the system after himself. But the "old" system depicted on the right side of the chart shows only Wu Jianquan defecting from the traditional Yang style. Jianquan was taught by his father, Wu Quanyu, himself taught by Yang Banhou. This Wu system became popular in Hong Kong and southeast Asia.

All of the above lineage details are simply to show the change occurring in taiji over time and in major systems. And there was no end to it on the individual level. Yang Chengfu, in the preface to his *Taichi T'i-yung Ch'uan-shu* [Complete principles and applications of taiji, 1934], wrote that, looking back at photographs made ten years earlier, he saw that his old postures were inferior to those of the new ones (Wile, 1983: 155). In the interim, Yang had grown obese and no longer had the flexibility in left bow-step to turn his waist leftward to the front and to turn his back right foot leftward forty-five degrees from ninety degrees. And yet, looking at the photographs, one readily agrees with Yang: although he had grown fatter, his postures are superior to the old ones.

When the spirit hit him, Professor Zheng would show a few variations for certain postures. In fact, in New York City he taught diagonal flying as a more open posture, with the left arm raised and stretched out leftward like a bird's wing opening, instead of keeping it just outside the left thigh. This and other nuances may have been a factor in some New Yorkers claiming that they had received the "fully evolved form" (an assertion they sometimes used to counter the Taiwan old-timers' contention that Professor Zheng taught them the real form but had diluted it later for "lazy" Americans).

Sutton errs in contrasting the Yang 70/30% front-loaded bow step with the "Zheng" 100/0% (rounded off from his 99.9/0.1%) (1994: 59). Sutton should have asked himself why Professor Zheng would teach the bow step, front-loaded weighting as 70/30% all of his life (see the foot-weighting diagrams in all his books) and then a year or so before his death change it to 100/0% for his last student, Wu Guozhong. The short answer is that Professor Zheng did not change the weighting.

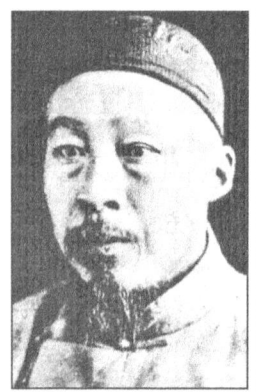 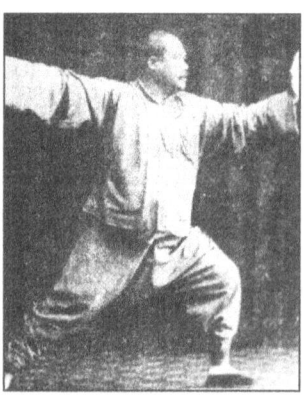 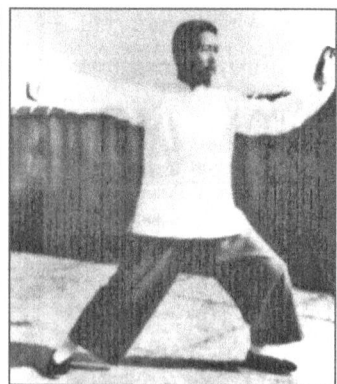

Left: Chen Weiming. Single-whip postures of Yang Chengfu (center), ca. 1933 and Zheng Manqing, ca. 1948.

In our collaboration, *T'ai-Chi*, I asked Professor Zheng whether auxiliary exercises to enhance correct breathing, the postures, and overall agility were beneficial. He responded that the postures themselves are so fully founded, variable, and beneficial that additional exercises would only detract from a student's progress. Sutton's assertion that Professor Zheng taught a range of auxiliary exercises for the development of neigong, exercises regarded as coming from the Zuo Laipeng system, is, therefore, inaccurate (1994: 59). Zheng was a quick study and if he concentrated on a thing he would have it. He was an encyclopedia of the esoteric, the ultimate dilettante in the best sense. He tried a myriad of neigong methods and, if he added the variable of time to concentration, he got a thing good. No one around today knows what he learned from Zuo Laipeng, but Zheng was impressed with Zuo's wisdom as imparted by Zhang Qinlin, from whom he probably received Zuo's teachings as well.

But in his preface to Zheng Manqing's *Thirteen Treatises*, Chen Weiming writes that, after Zheng arrived in Sichuan (1939), "[H]e met an extraordinary man, studied with him, and made great progress" (Wile, 1985: 1). Chen was close to Zheng and knew that he had an uncanny ability to attract great men wherever he went. Thus, this may mean that—even for Zheng—the Sichuan man was exceptional. Professor Zheng never noted the man by name, unusual perhaps for someone who had helped him progress. Could it have been Zhang Qinlin or even Zuo Laipeng relocating, as Zheng had, westward away from the invading Japanese? Ben Lo believes that Zheng stayed in Shanxi during World War II, but we do not know for sure. It remains a puzzlement.

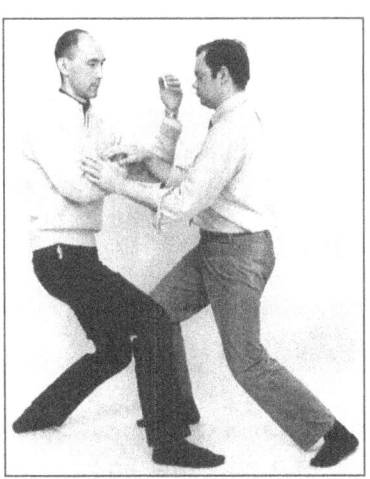

Tam Gibbs (right) doing push-hands
with Ed Young in New York City.

Professor Zheng was often jocular and during such moods would often show snatches of neigong, but he believed that students are easily diverted into laziness and wanted to have them use their time in taiji itself. Late in life he did develop "eight methods," a splendid set for older people. He did not teach it in a regular class, but I learned half of it from Tam Gibbs before his death and of this I retain the slenderest memory. In New York City, he taught several massage methods and ways of nurturing qi, and these can be learned from Wolfe Lowenthal's insightful first book on Professor Zheng, *There Are No Secrets* (1991: 112–122).

I never met Yue Shuting, Lu Tongbao, and Li Beilei, leaders of the second of three streams of Professor Zheng's teaching in Malaysia, nor did Zheng ever mention them to me (he did speak favorably of Huang Xingxian). I have heard from a reliable source that Yue's lungs were affected by wounds he received from the Japanese in World War II. If what Sutton writes of Yue's group is true, however, I shake my head sadly. He writes that they had a more muscular taiji than Huang Xingxian, that they prevailed in tournaments, and that Mr. Lu was known for sparring with and beating up his students (1994: 63–64).

Let us take these in order. Muscular taiji, like free love, is a contradiction in terms. Zheng Manqing taught that there was no hard in taiji—only different degrees of soft. Echoing Yang Chengfu, Chen Weiming wrote, "Those people who say you must use force usually have excess strength or practice with a hard style and won't give it up, thus never obtain the essence of taiji" (Lo & Smith, 1985: 18), and again, "People using force cannot benefit from taichi . . . they have failed to internalize the art" (Lo & Smith, 1994: 42). Professor Zheng wrote that we must "completely spurn muscular force" and that we should "relax completely and not exert muscular force" (Cheng, 1962: 13). It seems unlikely that anyone who would stress a more muscular taiji is practicing the taiji of Professor Zheng.

The fact that the Yue stream won more tournaments suggests a correlation between muscle and tournaments that should make Sutton pause. Tournaments are anathema to taiji. I have seen several. I cannot remember ever seeing relaxation there—only tension and force.

Taiji, to the extent that it becomes commercial and overly competitive, is no longer the real taiji that Chen Weiming loved so well. After all, taiji comes from Daoism which opposes all competition. Moreover, push-hands is meant to be a quiet means of testing and confirming one's form with another person while adhering to the basic principle established centuries ago of "no resistance and no letting go." Push-hands is not for commerce and ego. This principle was violated by Mr. Lu's sparring with and beating up students. I don't know what Sutton means by this, but it smacks of something other than taiji.

Some critics, Sutton writes, believe that taiji is presently weak because

Professor Zheng's first generation of students in Taiwan were mainly intellectuals and academics (1994: 59). Who asserts this and what is the evidence? Sutton should give such critics a wide berth.

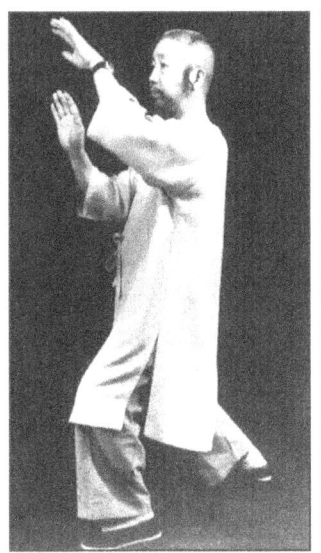 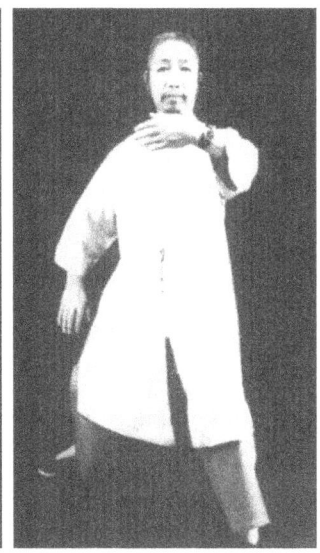 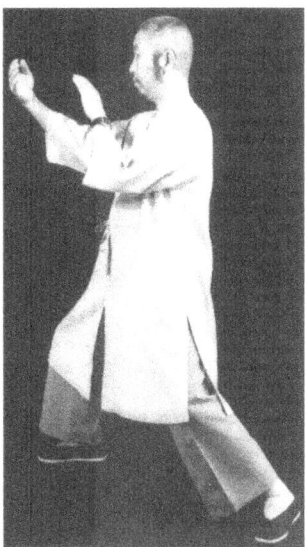

Zheng Manqing in lady works at shuttles, ward-off, and rollback.

In fact, contemporary taiji is vibrant and hardy. Thousands of people everywhere have better health and a richer life thanks to Professor Zheng's taiji. Today, it is strong—and getting stronger—in substance and spirit. True, many gentry were drawn to him by his Olympian accomplishments. But he accepted people from every station of life (in New York City, he had problems with local Chinese because he flung open his door and heart to the hippies of that time). Even if the contention that he taught the elite were true, there is no correlation between gentry and weak taiji. I think Sutton is talking of "tournament taiji" and muscular push-hands, which are not taiji at all. He must read again the *Classics* and *Zheng's Thirteen Treatises*, both of which condemn muscularity. For myself, I think the ideal student for push-hands is a person with little or no athletic background whatsoever.

When Sutton writes that Zheng Manqing, while trying to promote the cultural aspects of his art, "recruited" most of his top students by beating them in challenges of one form or another, he is being too sanguinary (1994: 62). The verb "recruited" should be deleted—Zheng did not have to recruit anyone—and "challenges" ought to be softened. Probably most challenges were simply push-hands tests in which the outsider found no place for push or pull and, at once enthralled by Zheng's body brilliance and frustrated by his own ineptitude against it, just gave up.

I say this with some understanding. When Professor Zheng came to New York City in the 1960s, I visited his studio frequently. On my first visit, in the midst of a lecture, he called me to the front and introduced me to the class as a boxer who had travelled around southeast Asia challenging all and sundry. This was not quite so. I did seek out taiji teachers for push-hands and got on famously with them, for courtesy and friendship prevailed. This does not mean that Zheng could not or would not wreak exquisite havoc if someone strayed outside the structured confines of push-hands (this too, I know from personal experience).

The point I am making is that Zheng was no gentle ruffian or thug. Sutton's bias toward muscular taiji would have bored Zheng. Whenever I or anyone else dwelled too long on combative matters, he invariably would start yawning, softly take the arm of the miscreant—often me—and blast him off the wall. True, he loved to talk with me about the Yangs, Du Xinwu, and other greats, but this was more in the historical rather than combative context.

Sutton's chief undoing, I think, is that he believes too much of the gossip, forever rife, in boxing circles. For example, he states that Professor Zheng's decision to leave Taiwan for the US in the midsixties was not made for altruistic reasons or to share his art with the world (1994: 60). But then he does not drop the other shoe; he neglects to tell us why Zheng went. I had spoken with Professor Zheng about a trip to the West shortly before I returned to the US from Taiwan in 1962, during the Cuban missile crisis. He went in January, 1964, to show his art at the Cernuschi Museum in Paris; he was the first artist ever to give a one-man show in the fifty-year history of that institution. This show was followed the same year by a one-man show at the World's Fair in New York, in 1968 at the FAR Gallery in New York, and in 1973 at the Hudson River Museum. All these shows met with lavish critical praise. Professor Zheng was honored but had to take out a bank loan to cover expenses for the first show. I only learned of the loan recently. It says something for his altruism that he never asked his students to support the trip financially, which all of us would have done without a second thought. On the way home from Paris in 1964, Zheng visited old friends and made new friends in New York City—artists, literati, and taiji aficionados—many of whom urged him to relocate here and promised him support. In due course he accepted. In any case, it strikes me as journalistically unethical on Sutton's part to claim to "know" something bad about a person and indict him with a hint and wink, but never name the fault.

Sutton ends his article by criticizing Zheng Manqing for being abstract on function, quoting from *Thirteen Treatises*: "If one is able to interpret energy and master the techniques, one's applications will be successful" (1994: 70),[11] then complains that Zheng does not reveal exactly how to interpret energy and master the techniques. But he does. He tells us continually in his writing and teaching to persevere in the postures and push-hands and to follow the basic principles of the *Classics* faithfully with belief, to become familiar with correct touch, to learn listening energy (*ting jin*), and to gradually comprehend interpreting energy (*dong jin*). Some of these lessons are provided in the very chapter from which Sutton quotes (Lo & Inn, 1985: 204).

No other person in taiji history has shed so much light on the more esoteric aspects of the art as has Zheng Manqing. When he first published *Thirteen Treatises* in 1950, he even wrote a series of articles in the major newspaper in Taibei telling his all-Chinese audience how to understand the more arcane subject matter in the book.

Zheng said he could not give us a pill (they don't make pills like that). Taiji is a microcosm of life. One has to work at it and work hard, through its agonies and exultations, and only then will it yield its favors. Why else did Zheng say that, of all his excellences, taiji was the most difficult? So, though his words can guide us and help us, they cannot do our job for us nor even fully help us understand it. Confucius said, "When I have presented one corner of a subject to anyone and he cannot from it learn the other three, I do not repeat the lesson" (Legge, n.d.: 203).

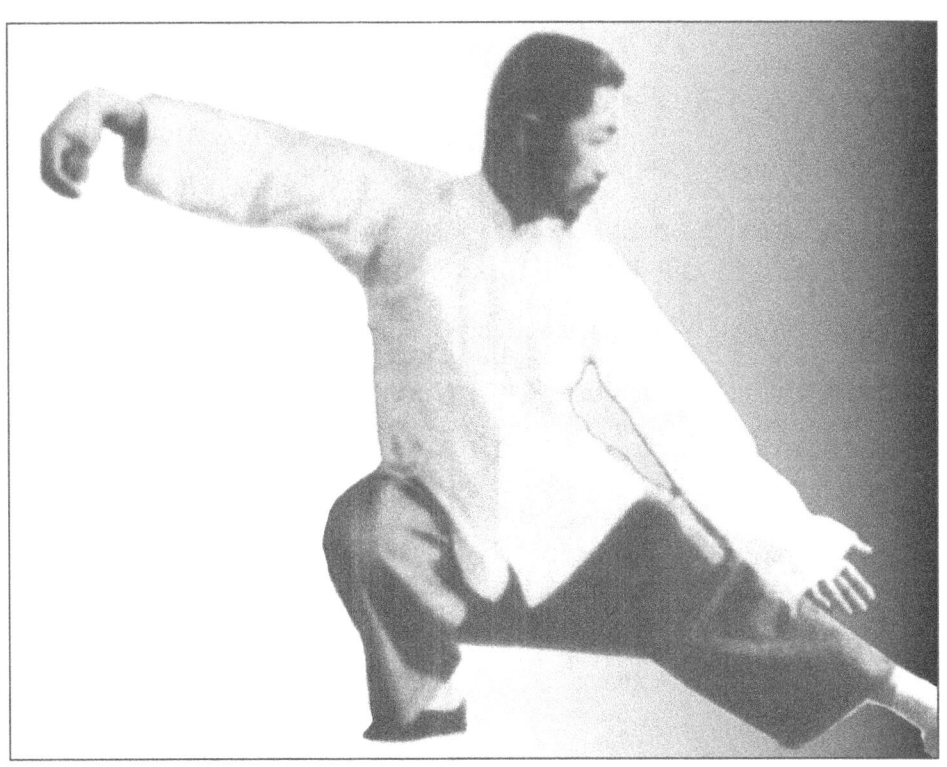

Squatting single whip, ca. 1948.

Professor Zheng, while alive, was often the target of gossip by inferior boxers, largely in Asia. Envy is a great stimulus. The villains, "boxers of the mouth corners," had only to approach him to be educated, but they avoided the opportunity like Dracula did garlic. Now that he is dead, it is worse—Zheng's own students sometimes behave poorly out of egotism. This is a shame. Add to which he is accused of keeping secrets by a writer who will not read or consult,[12] apparently cannot understand, and whose attitude cries out for infinitely more practice in "quiet minding." Put simply, Professor Zheng stood for good. I hope Mr. Sutton can come to see this.[13] In writing to protect Professor Zheng's estimable name, I am no sycophant, but just a person who wants to right a wrong. Here I have tried to "use all gently" (as the Bard says). But if Mr. Sutton finds my words harsh or in need of corrigenda, he should let me know so that I can correct them.

Transliteration of Chinese

Wade-Giles	Pinyin	Wade-Giles	Pinyin
PEOPLE		Wu Yu-hsiang	Wu Yuxiang
Chang Ch'in-lin	Zhang Qinlin	Yang Pan-hou	Yang Banhou
Ch'en Ch'ing-ping	Chen Qingping	Yang Ch'eng-fu	Yang Chengfu
Ch'en Wei-ming	Chen Weiming	Yang Chien-hou	Yang Jianhou
Cheng Man-ch'ing	Zheng Manqing	Yang Lu-ch'an	Yang Luchan
Han Yu	Han Yu	Yang Shao-hou	Yang Shaohou
Hao Wei-chen	Hao Weichen		
Huang Hsing-hsien	Huang Xingxian	**PLACES**	
Li I-yü	Li Yiyu	Pei ching	Beijing
Liu Hsi-heng	Liu Xiheng	Ch'en-chia-kou	Chenjiagou
Lu Tung-pao	Lu Dongbao	Nan ching	Nanjing
Sun Lu-t'ang	Sun Lutang	Shanshi	Shanxi
Tso Lai-p'eng	Zuo Laipeng	Szechwan	Sichuan
Tu Hsin-wu	Du Xinwu	T'aiyüan	Taiyuan
Tung Ying-chih	Dong Yingjie		
Wan Lai-sheng	Wan Laisheng	**PRACTICES**	
Wang Tsung-yueh	Wang Zongyue	nei-kung	neigong
Wang Yan-mian	Wang Yennien	t'ai chi ch'üan	taijiquan
Wu Chien-ch'uan	Wu Jianquan	t'ai chi shih-i	taiji shi yi
Wu Ch'uan-yu	Wu Quanyu	t'ing chin	ting jin
Wu Kuo-chung	Wu Guozhong	tung chin	dong jin
Wu Kung-tsao	Wu Gongzao		
Wu T'u-nan	Wu Tunan		

Notes

1. See page 57. In the first paragraph, the writer also suggests that the growth of taiji on the world stage is largely because of Zheng Manqing's style. This assertion can only be correct if one leaves out the influence of China itself with its millions of practitioners, relatively few of whom do the so-called Zheng style or even know of Zheng.
2. Wang Yannian recently wrote me correcting the year of the match from 1914 to 1924 (Julia Fairchild letter to R. Smith, October 16, 1994). Additionally, Liu Xiheng writes that a Mr. Hong, a student of Yang Chengfu who later lived in Hong Kong, saw the Zhang–Wan challenge match (letters to R. Smith, May 7 and 9, 1991). So the match occurred. But in *Chinese Boxing* (p. 38), I write that when Wan and Zhang squared off "the fight went nowhere: both injured their hands at the outset and it was postponed." The source for this was Zheng Manqing himself given orally to me. At the same time, he told me that earlier Wan had tested Yang Chengfu and was easily dispatched, saying as he left "two years" (meaning he would train for that period and return). When Wan challenged Yang again, Zhang intercepted. I tend to accept this version: Zheng knew both Yang and Zhang well and there was no need to slant the story. And it does not diminish Zhang—his glory days were ahead of him.
3. Wang Yannian inexplicably renders Zuo's given name as "Yifeng."
4. See page 38 of *Chinese Boxing*. The next sentence reads: "[Zheng] stayed with this man a while and derived a new method of doing the postures." I can't remember the source or even having written the sentence. The source certainly was not Zheng Manqing. I hope these words were not an ingredient in Wu Guozhong's claims. Lacking any corroboration for these words, since they were written over twenty years ago, I now disavow them.
5. Conversation with Wang Yannian in Bethesda, Maryland, September 24, 1984.
6. Letters from Liu Xiheng, May 7 and 9, 1991; Phone conversation with Ben Lo, August 1994.
7. See Tam Gibbs (1985). This article is dated November 2, 1978, and is an expansion of the memorial tablet largely written, according to Ben Lo, by Yao Menggu, an artist colleague of Professor Zheng. Gibbs fleshed out the text of the memorial for this article and his translation was done in the presence of Mrs. Zheng as she transliterated the classical language (*wen yen*) of the original into vernacular Chinese (*pai hua*) so that Gibbs could understand it and translate it into English.
8. Letters from Liu Xiheng, May 7 and 9, 1991.
9. Wu Jianquan's father, Wu Quanyu, was a top student of Yang Banhou.
10. I never met Wu Guozhong. A decade or so ago, he wrote me urging me to let

him put my name with his on a book he had written (presumably, the old Cheng-Smith nexus would then become Wu-Smith). The proposal struck me as strange, and I declined his offer.

[11] The writer incorrectly attributes this to Ben Lo and Martin Inn's translation of *Thirteen Treatises*, but the words are from D. Wile's *Advanced T'ai-chi Form Instructions*, p. 112. There is no substantive difference, however, in the two translations.

[12] Sutton should have consulted with me. If he had, many of these errors could have been avoided. He had erroneously stated that I made Professor Zheng's prowess known through the English-speaking world (p. 61). In this article and elsewhere, Sutton attributes Zheng's fame to my writing, confusing the message with the messenger. Let me be plain: Professor Zheng's reputation is the result of his extraordinary ability in taiji. His towering taiji earned him a deserved recognition. Sutton's error is the ultimate example, it seems to me, of confusing the teacher and the taught.

[13] Since Sutton is one of the few writers in the martial arts genre combining writing craft and style—and we must encourage such talent—it has been hard for me to criticize him. But the issues demanded it. Germanely, in passing, permit me to bow to karateka Graham Noble of England, who is able to bridge Eastern and Western martial arts in his facile writing; to Dave Lowry; to Canadian judoka Paul Nurse; to Hunter Armstrong, keeper of Donn Draeger's flame—who has that rare quality in the fighting genre—common sense. Last, but probably at the top of this short list, I would place the taiji teacher from Australia, Paul Lynch, whose writing stands and moves and is always lubricated by intelligence and wit. With the advent of the *Journal of Asian Martial Arts*, I am sure this short list will become longer.

Bibliography

Cheng, M. (1962). *Taichi chuan: A calisthenics for health and self defense*. Taibei: Shih Chung Tai-chi Chuan Center.

Draeger, D., & Smith, R. (1980). *Comprehensive Asian fighting arts*. Tokyo: Kodansha.

Gibbs, T. (1985). Cheng Tzu: Master of Five Excellences. *Full circle*, 1 (2): 13–21.

Legge, J. (Trans.) (n.d.). The Confucian analects. In *The four books*. Also in *The Chinese classics*, vol. 1. Oxford: Clarendon Press (1893).

Lo, P., & Inn, M. (Trans.). (1985). *Cheng Tzu's thirteen treatises on t'ai chi ch'uan*. Richmond, California: North Atlantic Books.

Lo, P. (1985, August). Explanation of Tso-style t'ai chi ch'uan. *T'ai chi ch'uan*. Taibei: Taiwan.

Lo, P., Inn, M., Amacker, R., & Foe, S. (Trans.). (1979). *The essence of t'ai chi ch'uan: The literary tradition*. Richmond, California: North Atlantic Books.

Lo, P., & Smith, R. (Trans). (1985). *Ch'en Wei-ming, T'ai chi ch'uan ta wen* [Questions and answers on taijiquan]. Richmond, California: North Atlantic Books.

Lowenthal, W. (1991). *There are no secrets: Professor Cheng Man-ch'ing and his tai chi chuan*. Berkeley, California: North Atlantic Books.

Sutton, N. (1994). The development of Zheng Manqing taijiquan in Malaysia. *Journal of Asian martial arts*, 3(1): 56–71.

Wang Y. (1988). *Taijiquan*. Taibei, Taiwan: self-published.

Wile, D. (Comp. & Trans.). (1985). *Cheng Man-ch'ing advanced form instructions*. Brooklyn, New York: Sweet Ch'i Press.

Wile, D. (1983). (Trans.). *Master Cheng's thirteen chapters on t'ai-chi ch'uan*. Brooklyn, New York: Sweet Ch'i Press.

Wile, D. (1983). *T'ai chi touchstones: Yang family secret transmissions*. Brooklyn, New York: Sweet Ch'i Press.

Yang, C. (1975). *T'ai-chi ch'uan t'i-yung ch'uan shu*. [Complete principles and practice of t'ai-chi ch'uan]. Taibei: Chunghua wushu chupanshe.

Remembering Zheng Manqing: Some Sketches from His Life
by Robert W. Smith, M.A.

"Draw your chair up close to the edge of the precipice
and I'll tell you a story."
—F. Scott Fitzgerald

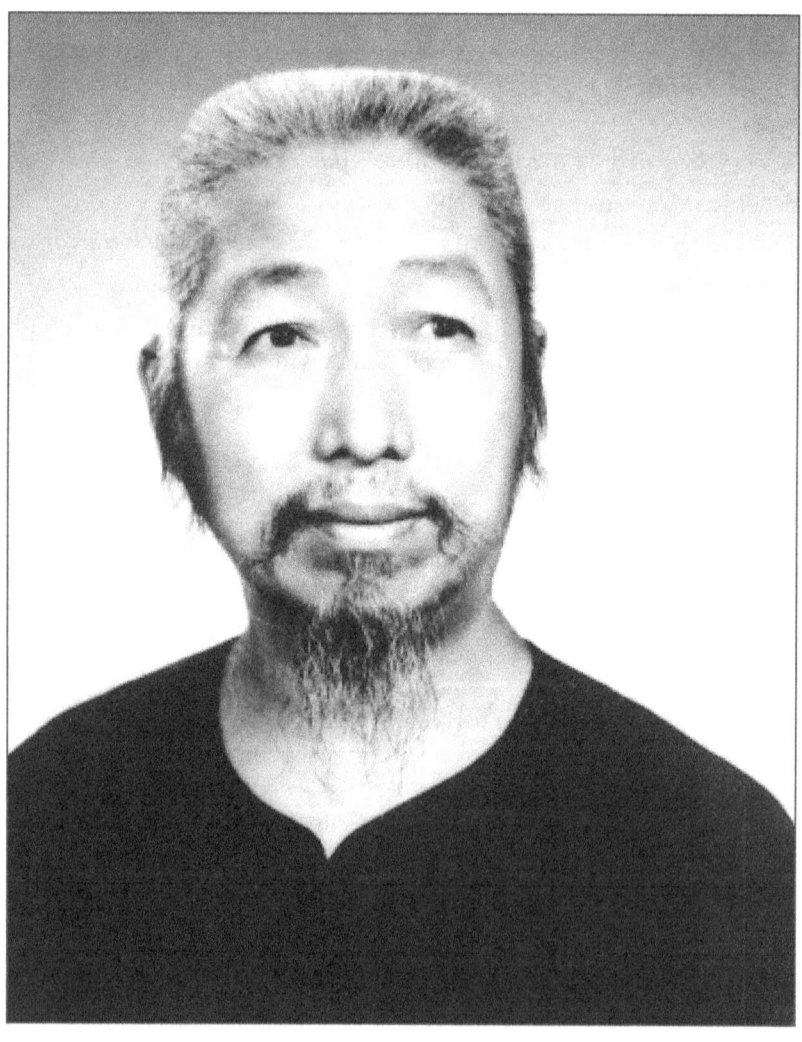

"I never wanted to become a Buddha;
I wanted to become a man." —Zheng Manqing
Photos courtesy of R. W. Smith except where noted.

Sometime after Professor Zheng died in 1975, Tam Gibbs, one of his senior taiji students, called me from New York City saying he had had an exhilarating talk with Mrs. Zheng. He said in this discussion she described some events that occurred during the early years of her marriage to Zheng. A young, cultured woman—her father was a top figure in the Chinese Air Force—she was awed by the brilliance and energy of the forty-year-old Zheng. And often she didn't quite know what to make of his friends. She cited two boxers, man and wife, who would come to the Zheng home and never bother to knock at or open the outer gate—they simply jumped over it and strode in. Another boxer one night rose from his chair in the living room and bade her turn off the lights. She did. He then did a form in total darkness and all she could see were sparks and lights from his qi. When she turned the lights on and examined him for electrical sources, she found none.

Tam Gibbs urged me to interview Mrs. Zheng, saying I knew the history and liked a good story. I wrote her and suggested it. She politely declined, saying she was young then and her recall of names was so faulty that it would, she felt, negate the value of the story. She also owned that recalling the old days just then would trouble her emotionally. So I backed away.

Another of the stories she had told Tam that day concerned a young Western-style boxer, Guo Qinfang, the lightweight champion of China, who knew Professor Zheng well in the early 1940s. One day in Chongqing the Professor took Guo with him to see a "strange" boxer named Wang Xiuai.[1] When they got to the boxer's modest house, an emaciated man who looked like a coolie opened the door and politely invited them in. They sat down in chairs while the "coolie" huddled against the wall. After a little while, young, impatient Guo inquired of Zheng where the master was. Zheng pointed to the "coolie" and said, "That's him." Zheng spoke to the man and he answered. Zheng then told Guo to go stand before him, which Guo did. The boxer gently took Guo's hand, smiled, and without force—at least Guo felt no force, only an exquisite energy—put him facedown onto the floor. Guo got up and squared off with the man. No blows were struck, but the boxer suddenly appeared behind the stupefied Guo. The three then drank tea, talked awhile, and the visitors left, Zheng laughing, Guo enthralled but puzzled.

In 1992 I wrote Danny Emerick, studying under Liu Xiheng in Taiwan, and urged him to interview Mr. Guo. Sometime later, Danny sent me the manuscript of an interview in which he and translator Michael Schnapp, another longtime student of Liu, asked the questions to which Guo and, at one point, his boxing brother, Xu Yizhong, responded.

Guo Qinfang Meets Professor Zheng

"I [Guo Qinfang] first met Professor Zheng Manqing in 1930 at a Shanghai university. He was dean of the Chinese Arts Department, and I was attending one of his classes.

"Ten years later, during the war against Japan, I participated in a boxing match for the war effort against a 160-pound boxer named [Song] at Chongqing.[2] At the time I weighed 130 pounds. Since the bout was billed as an exhibition, I queried Song beforehand on how we should fight.

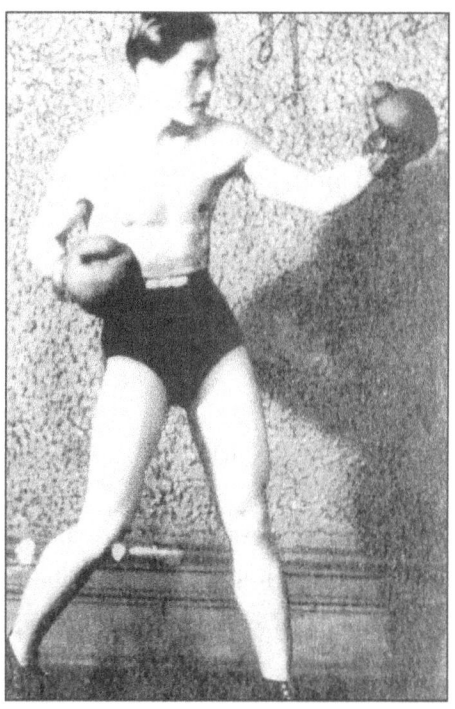

Guo Qinfang: Lightweight champion of China in the late 1930s. Photo courtesy of Guo Qinfang.

"'You'll see when we get into the ring,' he said curtly, letting me know that he was serious and not in an exhibition mood.

"In the first three-minute round we felt each other out and went to our corners to the sound of general hissing; clearly the audience wanted more action. Song responded by coming out for the second round with a barrage of blows. But I was ready and avoided his volley easily. In the third round, when he failed to react to a few of my jabs, I moved in with heavier punches to his head and soon he was hurt and hanging on. When he clinched, I concentrated my attack on his midsection.

"In the fourth round, because he hadn't connected once to my head, he went to my lower body. When this had no effect on me, he tried to hit me below the belt, bringing an avalanche of boos from the crowd and a stoppage of the fight by the referee. He left the ring forfeiting, and many in the crowd who had paid for six rounds demanded refunds. Trying to save the situation and his 'face,' I, the winner, told the crowd that Mr. Song had not violated the rules intentionally and that the money spent for tickets went to a good cause.

"Of course, I knew the low blows had been intentional. Later on, I learned that Mr. Song had moved to America and was famous for being 'the boxing champion of China.'

"It so happened that Professor Zheng was there watching the fight. He saw that Song had broken the rules and was concerned that I had been injured. He didn't know that I had been one of his many art students a decade before, but he thought my skill had been outstanding and sent Zhang Zigang, one of his senior students, around to talk with me. Zhang approached me, saying that his teacher really admired my gongfu and asked whether I had been hurt. I told him no, that I had dodged Song's punches and he had only hit my gloves. He said that his teacher would treat me if I liked. When I asked his teacher's name, he told me Zheng Manqing. I asked him what his teacher was and he said a doctor. I told him: 'Your teacher is my teacher and my teacher is a painter!'

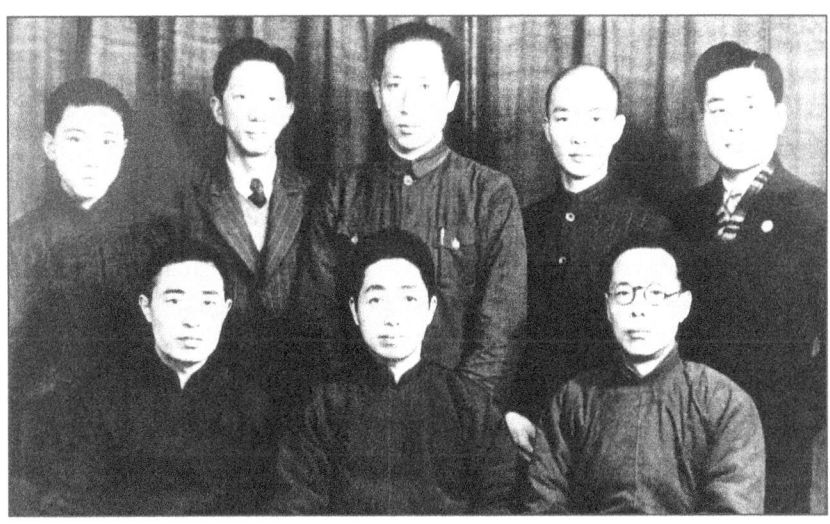

Photo of Zheng Manqing (center front), Guo Qinfang (rear row, far right with scarf), and Zhang Zigang (behind Zheng) in 1943. Others are unidentified. Zheng Manqing said Zhang probably was the most skilled taiji master on the mainland at that time.

"Later I studied taiji from Professor Zheng, but my main emphasis was still on boxing and how taiji could be applied to boxing, not quite the same as those who focused their energies solely on taiji. But with time, I was able to get a thorough understanding of Professor Zheng's teaching. When I box, I substitute for force his idea of overcoming the hard with the soft. I slip and duck my opponent's blows so that he can't land a single punch round after round. Of course, I'm speaking of head blows. I don't worry about body shots; special training has made me immune to these. But I never permit a head punch and so have never been injured there—unlike my teacher, Chinese Australian Chen Hanqiang ["Tacky"], an outstanding area pro of the 1920s and 1930s, whose ears were shifted out of place from head shots.

"When I teach a novice boxing, I first teach him to avoid and dodge so that he never takes a punch before I teach him to attack. If at first you teach him to attack rather than defend, he will be hit and will often become afraid. So, I teach him not to let himself get hit. This approach, of course, takes time and patience in the basics, such as jumping rope, hitting a ball or bag, and abdominal training so that you can take punches there. On the latter, you work until you can take just about any blow there. The abdomen can be trained in this way, but the head cannot. You can train only to avoid being hit but not to take punches to the head. If you take too many head blows, your brain will be damaged.

"Beyond this Western boxing training, I also was able to study some qigong. My teacher Huang in Chongqing was so versed in this mysterious art that [with permission] one could hit him in the head with a brick and it would have no effect. [In general practice] Huang would let anyone hit him anywhere except in the head—presumably, because of the eyes—without discomfort. One of his students, and a brother-student of mine, had practiced the art to such an extent that he would let a car run over his abdomen without injury.

"These abilities had more to do with qi than with muscular development. But there is another way: I trained, as I said before, with abdominal exercises. And this can be expanded to other parts of the body using a punching board. For instance, the lower arms can be trained by first hitting a wooden pole, starting lightly. Train until your arms become red, then purple, then black, and finally recover their original color. And then you are done—you then can take blows to the arms. In the end, you strike a steel pole. My students hit my arms, which are so hard that it hurts them. This is hard training and has nothing to do with technique. At first, you strike the pole twenty times progressing over time up to a hundred repetitions. Then you can work in pairs, striking each other's arms like this [demonstrating].

"One of Professor Zheng's students, the late Shi Shufang, has a special method of taking punches [Mr. Shi shows this ability in the 1960 film on Professor

Zheng made in Taiwan], and he once challenged me to an arm-striking contest. I told him I hadn't practiced this for a long time. He replied that he had challenged people all over the island and that there was no one who could beat him but that I shouldn't be afraid; after all, I was a famed boxer. I accepted and we went at it. After twenty or thirty of my strikes, he gave up.

"But he still would not accept defeat. He suggested slapping with the hands. When I was young, however, I had practiced 'steel-sand hand,' and so it took only ten or twelve of these exchanges before he surrendered. Steel-sand hand is so devastating that, once learned, it can never be used because the opponent's nose and head will bleed. I was supposed to train three years, but by the time I reached the halfway point I could not chance hitting anyone. In my painting practice, the brush in my hand began to feel like a nail, with no feel at all. So, I thought to myself: 'This is wrong. My hands are numb—what good is it? Even as a fighting tool, it is too terrible, impossible to use without inflicting serious injury.' So, I told my students not to train this way.

"In steel-sand practice, you really use steel sand, but you start with green peas and add the steel sand later. I was able to use this open-hand tactic against an opponent's arm in boxing as a block, but, of course, it was illegal against the head.

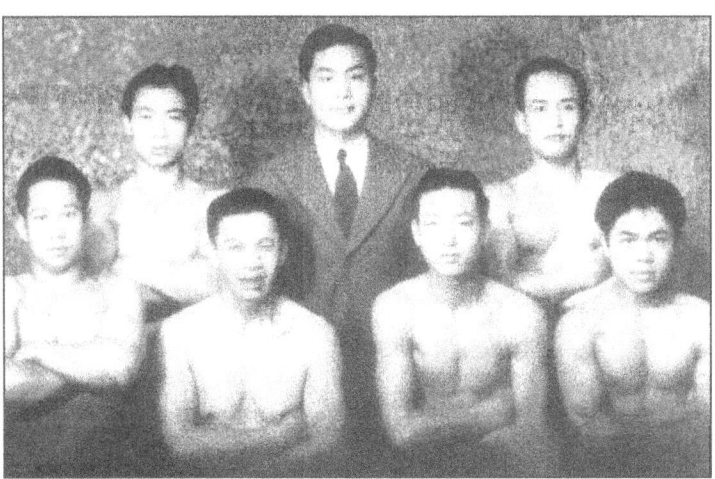

Guo Qinfang with the Jing Wu Boxing Team on occasion of his win over Topolesky, the Russian lightweight champion, at the 1937 International Boxing Tournament in Shanghai. Guo is suited and standing in the middle of the group. Seated in the first row, second from left, is Cheng Hanqiang (Tacky Chen). Seated fourth from left is Guo Huitang. Standing on the left of Guo is Pan Guohu. The identities of the others in the group are unknown. Photo courtesy of Guo Qinfang.

"Coming back to Professor Zheng, he was always studying many things. While we called him our teacher, he had people whom he called teacher. One, especially gifted, was the man who led warlord Feng Yuxiang's broadsword troop. Once, when I went to the Professor's house, he was upstairs practicing a method of this man's. When he came down, I asked what he'd been doing and he responded, 'Practicing *dianxue* [the art of attacking vital points].' This art was closely held and few would be taught its secrets. Zheng Manqing's maternal aunt, Hong Lei, said that the adept who headed the famed broadsword troop—I've forgotten his name—used to be rather short but suddenly grew taller when he got married. I asked how this could be and she replied that he used to be very heavy and liked to practice *qing gong* [light gongfu]. He became superb at jumping skills, leaping over walls and onto roofs. He would sleep hanging vertically on a wall in a hammock. So his heaviness and spurt in height might have been a result of this. One time, three men simultaneously attacked him. Two immediately fell and one ran away. Oh, his gongfu was exceptional! At the time, the Professor's aunt introduced them and he began to teach the Professor. This adept was about fifty.

"Occasionally, Laoshi [Since he taught at a university and was a taiji instructor, the titles of "Laoshi" (teacher) and "Professor" are often used when talking about Zheng Manqing] would call me over and say, 'Young Guo, let's play a bit.' But I knew all he had to do was to get me once on a vital point and it would be over. And, at this time, he'd only learned to attack points, not how to cure the results of an attack. So, I would tell Laoshi that, if we put on boxing gloves, I would be willing to 'play.' But I wasn't willing to play empty handed. Therefore he would often test my gongfu wearing boxing gloves, and every time there was a boxing exhibition at the British Embassy he would take me along.

"One couldn't tell many of the great boxers of the past simply by their appearance. I often admonished my students at Shi Da [Shi Fan University] that they should not take what I taught them to the streets and get into fights. You can never tell who has gongfu. You may think that an old guy on the street may be easy to bully, but the moment you act, you find yourself on the ground injured. Even now, if someone starts to attack me, as soon as he makes a move, I sense it and my strike hits him before he hits me.

"The famous Du Xinwu mastered *qing* [light], *ying* [heavy], and Dao [Daoist] gongfu. Once in Chongqing, a friend he was visiting wanted to spar with him, but Du, then past eighty, declined, suggesting instead that each of them demonstrate some aspect of gongfu. For his part, Du showed qing by jumping onto the back of a chair and taking three steps with it. Then he sat down and rocked like this [demonstrating], but it was so difficult that his friend could not do it—only Du's bones could stand it.

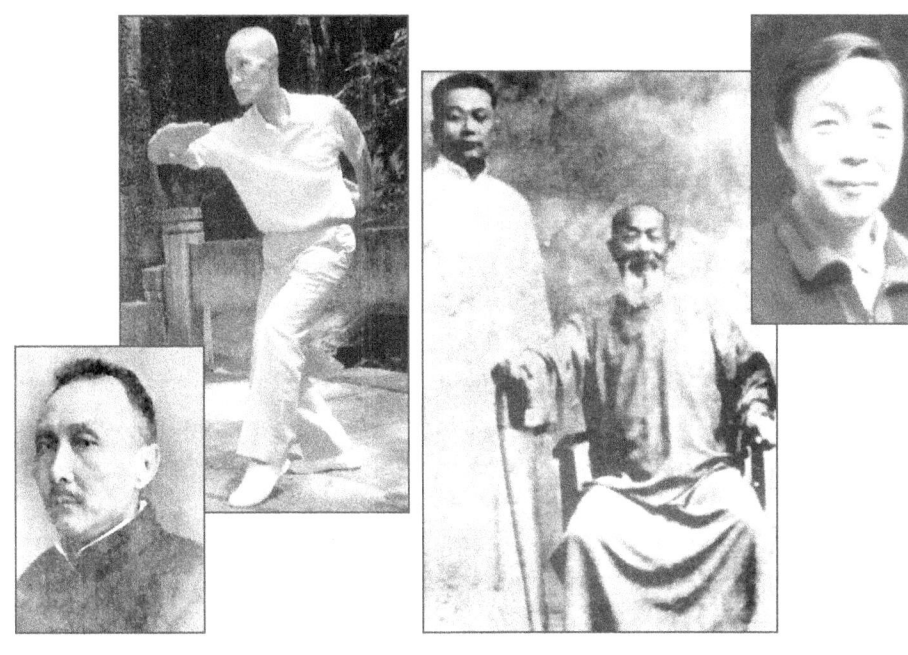

Left to right: Boxing legend Du Xinwu;
Wan Laisheng, protégé of Du Xinwu, whose
match with Zheng Manqing never occurred;
Wu Mengxia, who beat Wan but not Zheng to
the punch, with his *bagua* teacher Gao Yisheng;
Xu Yizhong, a senior student of Zheng Manqing.

"Later, he went into seclusion in a Daoist temple in Hunan Province to practice the Dao. Zhang Shijun, a renowned doctor in Chongqing, was a student of Du and once went to visit the octogenarian former transport guard at the Hunan temple. When Dr. Zhang first arrived there, he couldn't see Du but, after a search, found him meditating in a corner. One of the students with Dr. Zhang put his hand under Du's nose and, horrified, found that Du was not breathing. He was dead. The other students with Dr. Zhang began crying, lamenting Du's passing. The lamentations stopped in about a half hour, when Du awoke to announce that he had been on a 'little trip.' In fact, he had been gone for eight to ten days and only came back then because of the commotion. As he came to and his paleness turned to pink and light returned to his eyes, his students asked him how he could still live without breathing for so long. He told them that he had not been breathing through his nose but rather through his abdomen. He seemed like a god able to go out on such trips. Of all the great ones I've seen or heard of, he was the most advanced."

Xu Yizhong Interpolates

"I've heard that once Du Xinwu sought out the young and talented Zheng Manqing. When Du asked Zheng to show his form, the brave Zheng demurred; he wanted to get right to the boxing. So they began. When Du attacked Zheng Laoshi, Zheng sat back into his rear leg, eliminating Du's energy. Feeling this, Du broke off, saying, 'Anyone who can fight on just one leg is really good!'"

[See Smith, 1974: 39, for comments on this match. Mr. Xu's account seems to give Professor Zheng the best of it. As I recall his words, however, Zheng told me that, when the elderly Du visited him, they ate, talked awhile, and then went to bed. In the middle of the night, Zheng was awakened by Du, who said, "Let's play awhile." Zheng got up and they went at it. Zheng said it was like an avalanche of softness: everywhere he turned, however he changed his posture, Du's foot was in his face. Obviously this was a friendly match, the strikes divorced from power. Zheng recalled that Du praised him for his ability to get into one leg, but, mainly, Zheng was saying he felt helpless in that blizzard of feet.]³

Guo Qinfang Continues

"Another famous taiji teacher was Li Huangze, so skilled in gongfu that he could drop a person from a distance without touching him. In push-hands, if you touched his arm, out you went. He had studied in Germany and was a college professor. I wanted to learn from him, but the war and my job situation prevented it. Once he pushed hands with a Mr. Yao, a corpulent *xingyi* adept. In the midst of the proceedings, that worthy launched a fist at Li. At this, Li took a couple of steps back as though he had been thrown away by the impact. When they stopped, Mr. Yao found some black spots on his body and realized he had been injured. These could have been caused by Li's use of mind [*yi*] rather than qi. Li, who not only had this 'touching' ability, but could also cure it, offered to do so. Instead, Mr. Yao went for treatment to Li's teacher, a woman, who had studied Buddhism in Tibet and combined that esoteric teaching with taiji. There are many mysterious things in China—things that can't be explained scientifically. These people worked diligently from their early years to master these methods. And they did not divulge their secrets easily. Even if offered large amounts of money by someone seeking to become a disciple, they would not accept the person unless he or she had an unblemished character."

[See Smith, 1974: 35. "I was there the day that the daughter of a former Chinese ambassador to the United States, a visiting taiji student, told Zheng Laoshi of Li Huangze, her taiji master in Shanghai. Zheng nodded that he knew the man. The woman then said that he had special powers. Zheng asked her to explain. She told how she had tired of push-hands and asked Li what he would do against a real attack. He urged her to attack. She attacked, but as she neared him a force propelled her back and she began bouncing up and down. When her feet began to hurt, she implored him to let her stop. With a pass of his hand, he permitted her to stop bouncing. She also said that, when he touched a student, his hands generated sparks. Zheng laughed at all this. 'I knew Li,' he said. 'His taiji was not too good. He could do the thing you mention, but only because you are a student. The trick will not work against an equal or a superior.' Zheng later told me that Li had learned taiji from Dong Yingjie (another senior student of Yang Chengfu) and subsequently had gained a special skill of 'knocking down without touching.' The skill depended on student awe, however, and would not work against a good boxer." I include this excerpt because of the interesting contrasting views on the same man by Zheng Laoshi and Mr. Guo. Essentially it was a matter of angle of slant: Zheng was looking down, Guo, up.]⁴

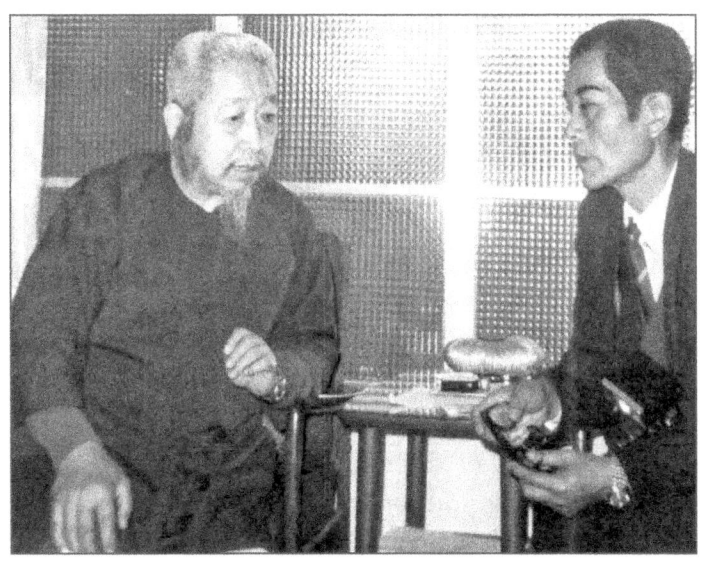

Two old friends talking. Zheng and Guo Qinfang
at Zheng's residence in Yungho, Taibei, 1968.
Photo courtesy of Guo Qinfang.

Mr. Xu Comments

"Doctor Hong Shihao was important in Zheng Laoshi's life. Hong is a ninety-two-year-old legal consultant—a Ph.D. from Harvard—who lives in Hong Kong and knows a lot about Zheng Laoshi's early years. I've seen him recently and he is quite healthy. When Laoshi left Beijing to teach at the university in Shanghai, Dr. Hong befriended him and took him to Yang Chengfu for taiji. When he first relocated south to Shanghai from Beijing, Yang had few students and it was Dr. Hong who brought him judges, lawyers, and other powerful people to learn taiji. Here Laoshi met Zhang Qinlin and others. Zhang himself had studied taiji elsewhere and his push-hands was excellent.

"Dr. Hong sponsored young Zheng. And when Dr. Hong came to class, Yang Chengfu would single out and teach Zheng more. But Hong was extremely busy with many foreign clients and, so, wasn't able to go to class all that often. Usually, Master Yang himself would not teach much; he stayed upstairs and let his son do the teaching. But when Dr. Hong came, Mrs. Yang would tell her husband he had arrived and Yang would go downstairs to teach. His students would then seize the opportunity to ask Master Yang about various aspects of taiji. Because Yang didn't teach much, his students behind his back would make remarks about him, such as saying that he was going to take his art into the coffin with him. But Zhang Qinlin had studied taiji and neigong [internal work] before he came to Master Yang, so often they would practice in the back. Zhang's gongfu was quite high and it was Professor Zheng's way to learn from anyone who was better than he was. Even though that person might be a brother of his, he would still call him 'laoshi.' So, Professor called Zhang 'Laoshi.'

"Wang Yannian, who lives here [Taiwan], studied under Zhang Qinlin on the mainland for a short time. So, when Wang first came to Taiwan, he visited Professor Zheng and told him he had also studied under Zhang; hence they were 'brothers.' That was really forcing it, but because Laoshi kindly called Wang 'classmate,' we then called him 'Uncle.'

"Now, another reason Master Yang gave Zheng Manqing special training was that Laoshi treated and cured Yang's wife of a debilitating illness. Thereafter, it was not only the influence of Mr. Hong, but that of the ever-present Mrs. Yang that ensured Zheng priority instruction. It helped also that he himself attacked the problems of taiji energetically and sopped up Yang's instruction like a sponge.

"Relaxation will bring good gongfu and also good health. In taiji we talk of 'body' and 'function.' The 'body' emphasizes health, and, of course, the 'function' stresses the martial side. Practice over time will enliven the body and reveal and refine fighting use. In taiji there is an advanced level in which I know that my opponent is going to use energy before he actually does, so I don't attack him. Only if he attacks will I respond and my counter will arrive first. Zheng Laoshi was outstanding in this kind of gongfu. [There is an apposite phrase in the *Classics*: "If my opponent does not move, I don't move either, but when he does I have already started moving and will arrive before he does."] Taiji also insists that it is the waist, not the hands, that moves. When you begin to understand what it means not to move your hands, then you have entered the door of the art."

Guo Qingfang Resumes

"Laoshi was really a good person, one always willing to learn from anyone more skilled than he and willing to teach anyone inferior in skill. Once, when I went to his house, I found him practicing a kind of gongfu that involved striking layers of tofu with a slender strip of bamboo held between his thumb and finger. He mobilized his qi and tapped lightly against the top layer of tofu. After a while, when we looked at the tofu, it was unscathed, but when the top layer was removed, we saw that the bottom layer had turned to mush. Incredible! I don't know how he did it, but I'm sure it was genuine and not trickery. He put effort and energy into everything he did. When he set his mind on something, he wanted to become the best. And he was the best at many different things. If he could not be best at something, he would not even claim to be good at it. He was second best at a lot of things.[5] For instance, he was brilliant at Chinese-style chess. One time he played against the Chinese national grand champion and won two and lost three of the five games, but refused to be second best and so didn't pursue competitive chess any further.[6]

"Laoshi truly was an Olympian. Perhaps a superman. We've already told how intelligent he was, how quickly he could absorb something. This was his strong side. Everyone was in awe of his taiji. It made him famous. But he wouldn't teach just anyone. Based on a person's sincerity, he would decide whether or not to accept him as a student. With me, he sought me out because of my boxing skill. Now, I am his student. Good teachers are this way. They see natural ability in a person and they go out of their way to teach him or her without any condition. I'm that way with my students. It is sincerity, not money, that determines whether or what I teach.

"Once, Zheng Laoshi saw a classified ad in a newspaper about a man who claimed to have excellent gongfu—there was no match for him anywhere on earth. Zheng sought him out and announced that he had seen the ad and he would like to try him out. They squared off and one blow from Laoshi left the man with blood all over his face. This man had a reputation as a street fighter who liked to challenge gongfu types. Now, this local hoodlum had been beaten at his own game.

"I remember, too, a time in Chongqing when Laoshi was giving a demonstration for the American advisor group. He asked me to accompany him. To get from my office to his, I had to take a bus. While waiting in line, a fellow tried to cut in front of me. I told him that he had to get in line at the end. Suddenly he—pah!—threw a punch. I dodged slightly to the side while punching him at the same time. He fell to his knees. I told him that, since he broke the line, which was against the rules, I wasn't worried about him reporting the incident to the police. It turned out he was a plainclothes policeman, and, when we went to his unit, his superior said that I had hurt him. I replied that, if he were injured, I would be responsible for healing him. So, I went to Laoshi and told him about it, and he wrote a note telling the policeman that he was a doctor and would treat him for free.

"The next day, Zheng Laoshi was surprised when he examined the chap and found his jaw swollen on the side opposite to the one receiving the blow. The shock of the punch doubtless caused this. Laoshi asked him if he knew the man he had fought with and, when the man shook his head, Zheng told him that it was the boxing champion of China! Laoshi further told him that I had only used 50 percent; had I punched full force, his face would have been shattered. Notwithstanding this, the policeman still filed charges against me, but Zheng Laoshi quashed the charge. I felt sorry about the incident, of course, but when he threw that punch, I countered instinctively. It couldn't be helped."

Son Patrick Remembers His Father

In December 1989 I met with Professor Zheng's son, Patrick, a restaurateur and taiji teacher in Asheville, North Carolina, close to my home. After a tasty repast at his restaurant, he recalled some incidents that involved his father.

Recalling his childhood, Patrick said he and his brother Wayne often got into scrapes. Although his mother usually had the task of punishing the errant boys, occasionally his father would do it. But when he did, he invariably used a small stick and was careful never to use his hand when paddling his sons. Patrick learned later the reason that his father never used his hands to paddle them. It was simply too dangerous for Professor Zheng to use hands trained in dianxue (the art of attacking vital points) to punish his young sons.

Patrick's mother told him in 1992 that, when his father first joined the Yang Chengfu circle, the top student, Chen Weiming, was away for a time. When he returned, Master Yang introduced him to the newcomer and suggested they do some tuishou (push-hands). They did and, though Chen tried to push him, he couldn't find him. Young Zheng merely neutralized his every endeavor. Chen Weiming was greatly impressed and the two became close friends.

In Taibei one day, the pedicab in which his father and mother were riding was hit by an errant bicyclist. Professor Zheng reached up and flipped the bicycle and rider over so they couldn't hit Mrs. Zheng, who emerged unscathed. He, however, did suffer a small abrasion on one leg.

When Patrick was seven or eight, the Professor took him to an ancient master in southern Taiwan. The old man lived in a barnlike structure, and what really caught Patrick's attention on entering was a sword hanging from the ceiling, perhaps fifteen feet above them. This puzzled Patrick and he politely asked the oldster if the sword were his. When the master nodded, the young boy asked what it was doing in a place where no one could get it. The old man smiled and said, "Oh, I can get it," whereupon he rose into the air, hovered, got the sword, and brought it down so the boy could see it! As Richard Burton would say, "There ensued incredulity." Patrick acknowledges that if someone told him such a tale, he wouldn't believe it, but he has to—he saw it.[7]

A famed taiji teacher was coming down a gangplank from a boat when he was accosted by four bandits. Instantly he sent them sprawling. A renowned doctor and man of good will, he addressed the downed brigands individually: A, you see me in seven days; B, in fourteen; C, in a month; and D, in six months. They each became sick and came for treatment at the times he had specified. A taiji senior told me he knew this story and the teacher probably was Zhang Xiulin (died c. 1930), a master of taiji, bagua, and *dongpi*, a man about whom little is known. Zheng Laoshi mentioned him once to me, eyes bright, and said that he had not met him, but solid sources pronounced him "truly marvelous." So, this tale only concerns Zheng tangentially, as the teller.

When Patrick was managing a restaurant in New York City, he came down with a bad wisdom tooth. The dentist gave him five shots and had to break the tooth into four parts to get it out. His jaw was swollen and the pain so intense he couldn't sleep at night. Soon, he was a shambling wreck and went to his father for help. Laoshi began by telling him he had done right by letting the dentist do what he could and he, Laoshi, was interposing merely to manage the trauma. He told Patrick to sit in a chair and went behind him. Telling him to relax completely, he put his hand on Patrick's head and, in the time it took him to sense his father's hand, he was out. He woke the next morning miraculously refreshed and ready to take the medicine Laoshi had sent out for. The pain was gone. Patrick asked him, "Father, how did you do that?" to which Laoshi made a face as if to say, "It's much too deep to tell you."

I end with an occurrence relayed by Patrick to me from Mrs. Zheng in June 1993. This story still leaves me wondering. Mrs. Zheng told of attending an automatic-writing session with a woman friend and Tam Gibbs in Taibei after Laoshi's death in 1975. They entered a place where there was a sandy pit with a man seated at each corner. A seven-year-old girl held one end of a six-foot pole, and a male doctor in his thirties held the other end, effectively bisecting the square. A slender piece of wood was attached to the middle of the pole and hung down into the sand below. As questions were asked in Mandarin Chinese, the mediums—the girl and the man—held the pole lightly, and it responded by moving and, with its central wooden "arm," writing answers in Chinese characters in the sand. The four men at the corners—one of whom had lived in the US and was skeptical about the proceedings—transcribed the answers. After some general dialogue, Mrs. Zheng thought to test the mediums by switching to a Zhejiang dialect unknown to those there. The answers came back written in Zheng's unique "grass" writing, which she could read but the four transcribers could not. This shocked her greatly, as did what happened when she put a glass of his favorite cognac in the center of the sand. Without spilling a drop, the arm moved the cognac through the sand out of the way; it apparently was interfering with the writing! One of her questions, incidentally, was how Laoshi liked his favorite cognac. His answer: "Very much!" Other questions were on past events known only to the two of them.

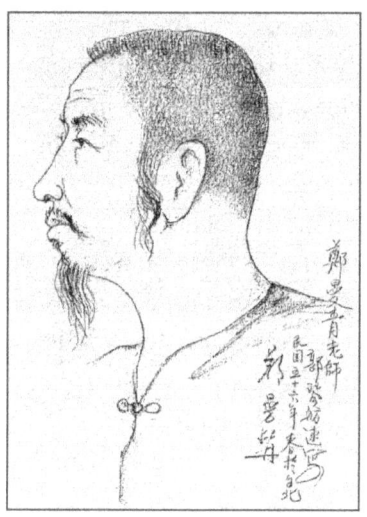

Teacher Zheng Manqing. Sketch by Guo Qinfang,
spring 1967. The Professor was so delighted at how
Mr. Guo had caught his spirit that he signed
the sketch himself. Courtesy of Guo Qinfang.

    I proffer no opinion on the authenticity of the proceedings, but would give a pretty penny to have been present. There was a popular craze (notice how those two words go together?) in automatic writing in England and America at the turn of the century, but much of it was fakery with questions limited to simple yes or no answers. This episode in Taibei, however, was not of that kind. It was, in fact, a full-fledged intimate conversation between a bereaved widow and her departed loved one. Readers must do their own mulling on this one. But enough! Though Mae West once quipped that "Too much of a good thing is wonderful," Confucius cautioned that we shouldn't talk too much, too loudly, or too often. There are other stories of this gifted, giving man, but they must await another time.[8]

Transliteration of Chinese

Wade-Giles	Pinyin	Wade-Giles	Pinyin
PEOPLE		Tung Ying-chih	Dong Yingjie
Chang Ch'in-lin	Zhang Qinlin	Wan Lai-sheng	Wan Laisheng
Chang Hsiu-lin	Zhang Xiulin	Wang Hsiu-ai	Wang Xiuai
Chang Shih-chun	Zhang Shijun	Wang Yen-nien	Wang Yannian
Chang Tze-kang	Zhang Zigang	Wu Meng-hsia	Wu Mengxia
Ch'en Han-ch'ing	Chen Hanqiang	Yang Ch'eng-fu	Yang Chengfu
Ch'en Wei-ming	Chen Weiming		
Cheng Man-ch'ing	Zheng Manqing	**PLACES**	
Feng Yu-hsiang	Feng Yuxiang	Chekiang	Zhejiang
Hsu I-chung	Xu Yizhong	Ching Wu	Qing Wu
Hung Lei	Hong Lei	Chungking	Chongqing
Hung Shih-hao	Hong Shihao	Hunan	Hunan
Kao I-sheng	Gao Yisheng	Pei Ching	Beijing
Kuo Ch'in-fang	Guo Qinfang	Szechwan	Sichuan
Kuo Hui-t'ang	Guo Huitang		
Li Huang-tse	Li Huangze	**PRACTICES**	
Liu Hsi-heng	Liu Xiheng	pakua	bagua
P'an Kuo-hua	Pan Guohua	hsing-i	xingyi
Shih Shu-fang	Shi Shufang	tien-hsueh	dianxue
Tu Hsin-wu	Du Xinwu	tung-pi	dongpi

Notes

[1] Conversation with Ben (Pangjeng) Lo, April 4, 1975. Tam Gibbs's version of this story was identical to Ben Lo's, but Mr. Lo was able to supply the name of this mystery man. Alone with Professor Zheng and Mrs. Zheng in New York City in the 1960s, Zheng told me about the great dianxue (vital points) teacher of this name he had trained under, but did not give the locale, and I assumed wrongly that this was one of two dianxue teachers he had studied with in Nanjing.

[2] Mr. Guo states that, in 1992 in a US martial arts magazine, the boxer he fought claimed to have TKO'd him. Despite this severely skewed account of the bout, since the boxer did not identify Guo by name, Mr. Guo believes he should accord him the same courtesy. So I call him "Song"—not his real name. Germanely, the *New Shu* (Shu is short for Sichuan Province) *Newspaper* of January 10, 1943, reporting on the boxing card of the day before, said, in part, "The highlight of the entire event was the match between Guo Qinfang and [Song], which was especially exciting. After four rounds, despite his smaller stature, Guo beat [Song] by virtue of his quick and agile movements" (translation by Michael Schnapp).

3   Wan Laisheng, a student of Du Xinwu, and Zheng Laoshi had an open challenge going through World War II, but they never clashed. I learned from Zheng himself that, at a party in Chongqing during the war, the host, famed Wu Mengxia, brought Wan Laisheng over to introduce him to Zheng and, while Zheng was warily watching Wan, host Wu lashed out at Zheng, who among the dropping teacups countered to Wu's eyes, momentarily blinding him. The defeated Wu specified "three years," meaning he would return in three years, but never did (see Smith, 1974: 37).

4   Professor Zheng told me in 1964 that Li Huangze, who had heard of Yang Chengfu from one of his math students, came to Yang and kowtowed seeking instruction. Yang said no, that he must kowtow to Dong Yingjie, who would be his student. Li did and later learned the special method.

5   Reminding one of Irish poet James Stephen's line describing Stephen Mackenna, that translator of Plotinus and greatest talker in Ireland: "He was wildly in love with everything he couldn't do." I was forever finding new arrows in Zheng's quiver. I visited the New York studio once to learn that someone had put a staff in his hands one day and he had taken the thing and trounced everyone there, repeating the course for some New York University fencers brought in a day or two later. There was simply no end to the man. This doesn't mean he was an overly competitive lout, but rather underscores his abiding interest in life and people.

6   Some experts informed me that Zheng was only second in certain arts—in calligraphy and as an authority on Laozi or Confucius, for instance. Other experts would dispute these assertions, putting him first, but even if true, a small catalog of seconds isn't bad. One thing was not in dispute. No one ever called him second in taiji.

7   Recalling Groucho Marx's classic quip, "Who do you believe—me or your eyes?" It is said that V. Nijinski, the greatest dancer the world has seen, did not levitate as some suggested. No, he leaped and what gave the appearance of levitation was that at the apex of the leap he hovered. This old man seeking his sword from on high had gravity against him and a boy's eyes and imagination for him. Obviously skilled in qing gong (light gongfu) he leaped high and got his sword, but he didn't hover. The boy's mind did that. But I could be wrong about this.

8   I can't resist a last story from Patrick Zheng deserving the rubric "strange" that concerns Professor Zheng's clothes. Laoshi designed his own clothes (he wouldn't wear a collar, the symbol of a slave in old China) and had them tailored by an old friend who didn't believe in machines and did all the work by hand. After Laoshi's death, his shade appeared to a senior student and asked why he hadn't been buried with an undershirt. When the student asked why he didn't

ask his widow, the shade said he didn't want to frighten her. So, the student sought an answer from Mrs. Zheng who, not knowing, asked the long-retired tailor who had made and fit all of Laoshi's coffin clothes. Puzzled, the tailor asked her, "How do you know about the undershirt? Only I know [that fact]." Then he explained that when he tried to put the undershirt on Laoshi, his body was so stiff it was too difficult to fit it on him. The tailor said he left it off, knowing no one would be aware of it anyhow. Someone apparently was.

Reference

Smith, R. (1974). *Chinese boxing: Masters and methods*. Tokyo: Kodansha International.

Acknowledgements

Thanks go to Guo Qinfang for wonderful help with the text and, especially, with the graphics. Michael Schnapp, Danny Emerick, Russ Mason, and Dan Johnston also had oars in the water. Messrs. Liu Xiheng and Xu Yizhong kept me from making too many errors. Lastly, I bow to Juliana Cheng and Patrick Cheng and also to Ben Lo, superb teacher and researcher on taiji, for his help in preparing this article.

Chen Weiming, Zheng Manqing, and the Difference between Strength and Intrinsic Energy
by Robert W. Smith, M.A.

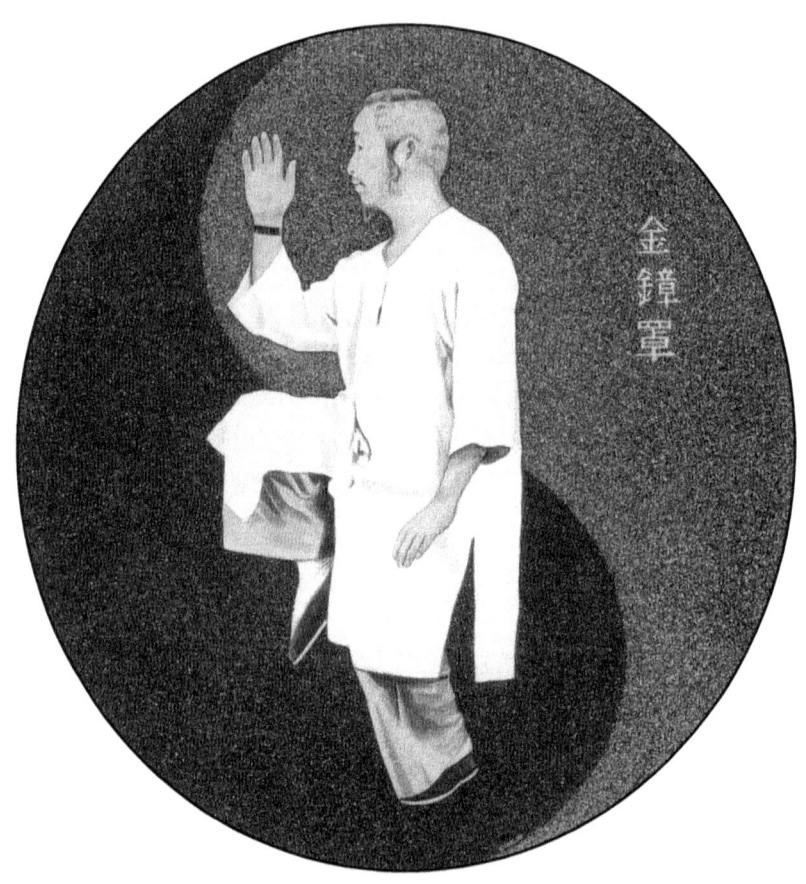

Zheng Manqing in rooster stands on one leg.
Illustration by Michael Lane.

When Zheng Manqing began learning taiji from Master Yang Chengfu in Shanghai during the early 1930s, he was a quick study. He had been practicing taiji with another teacher for two years and had conquered the tuberculosis that had been dogging him. At the same time, he learned to acquit himself well during push-hands with larger and more experienced students. This background provided him the impetus to soak up Master Yang's teaching like a sponge. Zheng's rapid progress accelerated even more after he treated and cured Mrs. Yang of a chronic malady, causing Master Yang to give him additional personal instruction.

During this early period, one of the most formidable of Master Yang's senior students, the scholar and writer Chen Weiming, was absent for a time on business. On his return, Master Yang introduced Chen to Zheng and suggested they try conclusions. Chen soon found the meaning of frustration. Every move he made, every push he tried, was unavailing. Newcomer Zheng neutralized him easily: Chen could touch Zheng but couldn't "find" a place on which to use his energy. This astounded the other students, who had stopped to watch, but not Master Yang, who knew young Zheng's ability even then. For his part, Chen Weiming, then near fifty, was impressed and immediately became fast friends with Zheng. The pair then became the intellectual leaders of Master Yang's group, cementing it and spreading the good news of taiji to the populace.

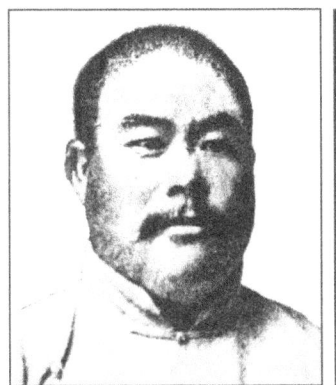 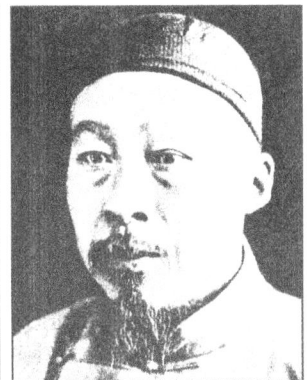 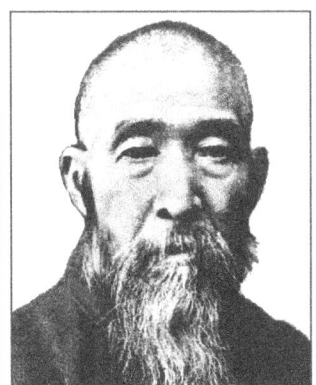

Left: Yang Chengfu, the taiji master. Center: Chen Weiming, taiji "older brother" of Zheng Manqing. Right: Sun Lutang, Chen's bagua teacher. Photos courtesy of R. W. Smith.

Chen Weiming Trains under Master Yang

Of all the great boxers Professor Zheng met during his life, none was closer to him than Chen Weiming (1881–1958). Chen came from a gifted family: his father was an intellectual, his mother was a calligrapher, and three of their sons passed the provincial examinations with high marks. Chen was employed by the Qing History Office and was esteemed by all who met him.

After moving north to Beijing from his home in Xishui, Hubei Province, in 1915, Chen began studying xingyi and bagua from famed Sun Lutang. Around 1918 he traveled to Hebei, where he went to the home of Yang Chengfu in Guangping County to ask Master Yang why, if his style of taiji were so good, he didn't teach it more.

Yang replied that he wanted to spread taiji and, since his grandfather Luchan had learned it from the Chens of Chenjiagou in Henan Province, he, Chengfu, would now repay the Chens by teaching Chen Weiming (Chen, 1925: preface).

Chen Moves to Shanghai

After training under Master Yang for seven years, Chen Weiming moved south to Shanghai. In 1925 he started the Achieving Softness Boxing Association (Zhi Rou Quan She) and wrote a book called *The Art of Taijiquan* [*Taijiquan shu*], which actually was a compilation of Master Yang's taiji teaching.

Chen's move to Shanghai was the first significant appearance of taiji in the south. Just as Yang Luchan had been the first to take the art to Beijing, Chen was the first to take the art to Shanghai. Qian Chongwei, who became one of Chen's leading students, describes his first meeting with Chen:

> Soon I saw a fair, elegant man enter the practice hall and sit on a couch at the side and watch everyone doing their postures. After a while he calmly got up and corrected them. I learned that this was Chen Weiming, the head of the society. I was surprised because I . . . expected that the head of a boxing group would be strong and vigorous, but Chen appeared to be an intellectual with a leisurely manner . . . . —Chen, 1927

Another of Chen's students, Hu Yunyu, learned taiji and sword from Chen for fifteen years. In a preface to Chen's *Taiji jian* [*Taiji Sword*], Hu admits to having learned a little, saying, "I am now past fifty and my body has gradually stiffened, a fact my heart and mind know and my tongue can say but, because of taiji and Teacher Chen, one that my body doesn't acknowledge" (Chen, 1927).

By 1929 taijiquan was well known in Shanghai and Chen's society prospered. After a time he invited Master Yang to visit. Whereas Yang previously had taught in a private or semiprivate venue, here he gradually opened taiji instruction to the public.[1] That same year Chen Weiming also helped his xingyi and bagua mentor Sun Lutang to relocate to Shanghai.[2] Meanwhile, Chen worked on books that stimulated the spread of taiji. Chen's *Art of Taijiquan* (1925) was followed in 1927 by *Taiji Sword*, and in 1929 by *Questions and Answers on Taiji Boxing* [*Taijiquan da wen*].

Once, while Master Yang was on a trip south, Chen's association brought Master Yang's "older brother" Yang Shaohou to teach for three months.[3] He taught the same large form as his "younger brother" during this time, but privately taught his idiosyncratic, small, trigger-force form too.[4]

Chen Recounts Stories of the Yang Family

In an appendix to his 1927 book *Taiji Sword*, Chen Weiming recorded the following:

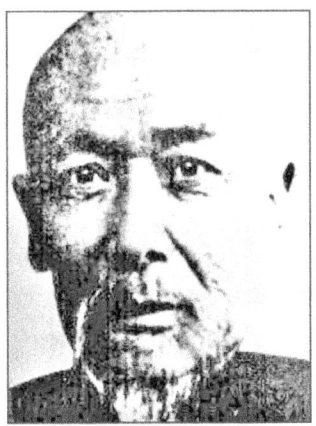

The painstaking and pains-giving Yang Shaohou.
Photo courtesy of R. W. Smith.

There are many schools of boxing, but only the Wudang school is pure *neijia* [inner family] handed down from Zhang Sanfeng.[5] One should use *qi* [internal energy], but not the slightest external force. Yang Luchan, a native of Guangping County in Hebei Province, first learned it from Chen Zhangxing of Chenjiagou in Henan Province. Yang later taught his sons Banhou and Jianhou. Later, Jianhou taught his sons Shaohou and Chengfu.

It came about this way. Yang Luchan first learned *weijia* [outer family]. But when he heard of the taiji skill of Chen Zhangxing, he sold everything and moved to Chenjiagou in Henan Province to study with him. For several years he practiced with the other students and was beaten soundly by many of them. But late one night, rising to go to the toilet, he heard a noise outside the wall. Peering through the window, he saw some of his classmates being taught secretly by Master Chen. After that, he covertly watched the class every night. The upshot was that one day the students asked him to push hands and he was able to roundly defeat them. They told Chen of this and he approached Yang, saying, "I've watched you for several years. You are honest and diligent. I will teach you the principles of real taiji. Come to see me tomorrow."

When Yang went the next day, Chen sat in a chair, apparently asleep or sick, his head lolling uncomfortably to one side. Yang, with his hands, supported Chen's head for a long time, and after a while, his arms ached from the effort. Finally, Chen appeared to awaken, noticed Yang, and told him to return the next day, as he was too tired to practice. Next day, Yang came again to find Chen apparently still asleep. When Chen awoke, he told Yang to return the next day. When Yang returned on the third day, Chen capitulated. "Very well, I'll teach you now. But you must practice in your room also." After this training, no one could stand before Yang.

Later, Chen assembled his students and scolded them. "I wanted to give my skill to you, but you couldn't get it. Yang was stronger and I didn't want him to get it, but he did. Now he is leaving."

From Chenjiagou, Yang went to Beijing to teach at the home of a rich family. The incumbent teacher there became angry at this intrusion and wanted to fight. Yang agreed but insisted that the master of the house should know first. When told, the master agreed but insisted that the bout be kept sportive rather than mortal. There was to be no killing.

They began. Yang took several steps and stood stock still. The other boxer quickly attacked and, just as quickly, was pushed several meters away. He acknowledged defeat by saluting Yang with a fist salute and they ate together. Immediately afterward Yang decamped, refusing to deprive the other of his job. He taught elsewhere in Beijing, being the first to introduce taiji there.

While gaining fame teaching others, Yang's real vigor was expended on his sons. He taught them many hours daily without stint. Both sons tried to escape, one to become a monk. Neither succeeded and by age twenty both were great experts. A member of the royal family invited Banhou to teach at forty dollars a month, a huge salary then.

In Song County of Hebei, there was a strong boxer surnamed Liu with over a thousand students. Some of these students started a friction between Liu and Banhou, and Liu challenged Banhou to . . . combat.[6] The whole city heard about it and thousands flocked to see the fight. Liu fiercely seized Banhou's wrist. (Yang later said it was like the bite of a dog.) Banhou used *jie jing* (a form of "receiving energy") and snapped his arm out of Liu's vise, causing Liu to fall heavily to the ground. Liu rose and hurried from the arena, while Banhou proudly strutted home to his father.[7] When he told his father of the bout, Yang Luchan smiled coldly and observed, "You did all right, I suppose, but your sleeve is torn off. Do you call this taiji energy?" After that, Banhou's fame spread but he was no longer proud.

Senior Fu Tells of His Experience

Yang Banhou's chief students in Beijing included Chen Xiufeng and Senior Fu. While Chen Weiming never met the former, he was able to visit Fu in Beijing. Though over seventy at the time, Fu looked fifty. In fact, his son, who was fifty, looked like his brother. Nevertheless, he told Chen that he could not teach Banhou's art because he had not taught or practiced it for more than forty years. Of his experiences, Fu said,

> My older brother was a good wrestler and he taught me some moves every day. Before he joined the army and went off to Gansu Province, he asked me to study wrestling diligently while he was away. Years later he returned and asked me if I had kept up my practice. I responded no, that I was studying taiji from Yang Banhou and that it would not be good to mix the strength of wrestling with the subtle energy of taiji. This so angered my brother that he struck at me powerfully. I quickly countered him with deflect downward, parry, and punch [*ban lan chui*] from taiji, and he fell out the door and into the yard. He couldn't get up for a while and took several weeks to recover. My father berated me and forbade me to practice taiji again. This was unfortunate but I had to obey.
>
> When I was young, Yang Luchan liked me for my hard work. Even after he was past eighty he practiced taiji every day. He often sat around smoking his long pipe and talking. I remember once he came to my door when it was raining and muddy. When he entered my house, though he had walked through the mire, his shoes were clean as new with no mud on them. This gongfu we called *ta xue wu hen* [to step on snow with no trace]. His son Banhou also had this ability but few knew this and I saw him do it only once.
>
> The day came when Yang Luchan wrote to all his disciples telling them that he was going on a trip and that he would like to see them before departing. They went to his house but their suspicions were aroused when they saw no carriage outside. Yang sat in the middle of the room so all could see and let each man take a turn at trimming his long pipe. For some time he advised and encouraged them in their pursuit of taiji principles. After a while he wiped his sleeve and passed away while sitting straight.

Yang Banhou also had "floating" gongfu. Away when his beloved seventeen-year-old daughter died, he hurried home to find her coffin nailed shut. He cried and became so agitated that he soared and was suspended eight feet up in the air, much to the astonishment of his disciples. I witnessed him do this gongfu, which we called *fei teng* [flying and soaring].

Chen Weiming Resumes

Banhou and his younger brother Jianhou were reluctant to show the art, believing that trouble follows fame. They were polite and never bellicose. One day a famed southern boxer came to visit Banhou, who was then past sixty. The boxer paid his respects and then, after some friendly words, asked if it were true that Banhou had sticking energy [*zhan*]. Modestly, Banhou said, "My father had this skill. I know a little about it but certainly don't have his skill." The boxer would not be put off and persisted. Banhou asked how he wanted to test him. The visitor suggested that they put bricks two feet apart in a circle and [said], "I will get on the bricks and you follow with your right hand attached to my back. If your feet leave the bricks or your hand leaves my back, you lose."

Banhou agreed: "Very well. I am old and apt to get dizzy, but since you ask, I will do my best." On the bricks, the boxer began slowly and Banhou followed, concentrating his spirit. The man accelerated and suddenly his body became like a swallow, exquisitely light, and Banhou had to use his "flying" skill to keep up. But try as he might, the man couldn't rid himself of Banhou's hand. Finally, with one quick movement, the man jumped to the roof and turned around to find Banhou gone, leaving no trace. The boxer turned again and there was Banhou, his hand still on the boxer's back. "Let's get down," Banhou said. "You've made me very tired."

Yang Luchan's youngest son, Jianhou, once taught taiji at a military compound. One day, returning there from town, a local strongman attacked him with a club from behind. Jianhou easily deflected the attack and pushed the man ten feet away. Indeed, Jianhou was so skilled he would let a swallow stand on his open hand and prevent it from flying off. Incredibly, Jianhou would "hear" its tiny energy and yield so that the bird would not have the needed base from which to initiate flight.

Yang Luchan's disciple, Wang Lanting, also had great ability, but, alas, died early. Li Binfu, Wang's senior student, inherited a part of his art. Once a robust young boxer from the south visited Li and challenged him. The boxer had qigong skill and could move chairs and tables without physically touching them. Li, holding a small dog in his left arm, tried to refuse, but the boxer attacked him, giving him no time. He did have time, however, to deftly knock the youth down while not relinquishing his gentle hold on his dog. The southern boxer cried bitterly and left.

I learned taiji from Yang Chengfu for several years. He said: "One must distinguish the pure from the motley. Many practice taiji nowadays, but it is not the real taiji. The real has a different taste, and is easily distinguished. With real taiji, your arm is like iron wrapped with cotton. It is soft and yet feels heavy to someone trying to support it. You can feel this in push-hands practice. When you touch an opponent, your hands are soft and light but he cannot get rid of them. When you attack, it is like a bullet penetrating cleanly and sharply [*gan cui*], yet without using any force. When he is pushed ten feet away, he feels a little movement, but no strength and no pain. In touching him, you don't grab him. Instead you lightly adhere to him so that he can't escape. Soon his two arms become so sore he can't stand it. This is real taiji. If you use force, you may move him. But it will not be clean and sharp. If he tries to use force to hold or control you, it is like trying to catch the wind or shadows. Everywhere is empty. It can be likened to walking on gourds on the water. You cannot get to where the substantial is. Put simply, real taiji is marvelous.

A Word on the Photographs in Chen's First Book

Because the taiji form photos in Chen Weiming's *Art of Taijiquan* raise questions, let me venture some modest opinions. These photos include fifty pictures of Masters Yang and Chen doing postures, four of Master Yang doing push-hands and *dalü* (large rollback) with Xu Yusheng, and nine of Chen Weiming doing push-hands and dalü with Chen Zhijin (Chen, 1925).[8]

Obviously, not too much can (or should) be made of still photos, and I have chided some westerners for using them to draw sweeping conclusions. But perhaps this needs saying anyway, since these photos puzzled me greatly when I first saw them in Taiwan in 1960. When I asked Professor Zheng about them, he replied that photography was a new and rare thing in China during the twenties and that it took a while for taiji teachers to understand how to use the medium correctly.[9] One senior even suggested Yang and Chen had purposely posed incorrectly so casual readers would not get the real taiji as personal students did. While the same things are said about masters of karate and many other martial arts, I personally doubt this.

Therefore, let's look at these graphics in which both Yang and Chen are doing the same form but, shall we say, differently. First, Yang and Chen both do exceptionally long and deep postures. This is especially noticeable for the smaller Chen, who would have had trouble separating his weight in such low stances. Often both of their backs appear slightly bent, their rear legs fairly straight, and their wrists "broken." Yang often thrusts his chin out, and though better, Chen's head is also awry at times. In bow posture, both turn their rear toes only slightly inward from ninety degrees.

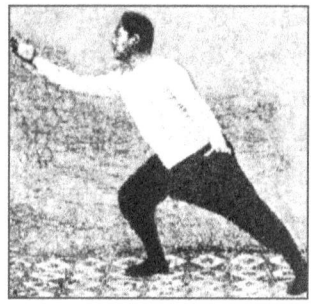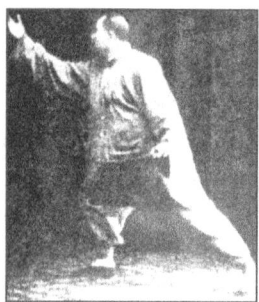

In the early photo (ca. 1918) of diagonal flying,
Yang is not erect and his rear leg is locked.
In the later photo (ca. 1932), Yang stands straighter,
his left knee is bent a bit, and he appears more relaxed.

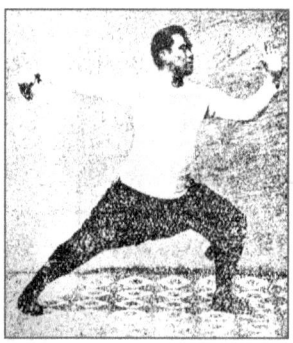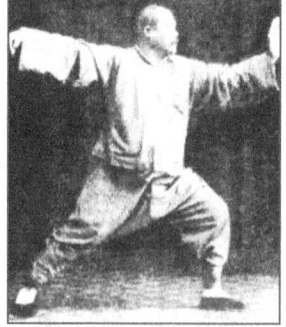

In single whip, Yang's posture is longer—and stiffer—
than the relaxed later one. Although deeper, Yang in
the early shot turns his rear foot slightly inward from
ninety degrees but keeps it at ninety degrees in the later one.

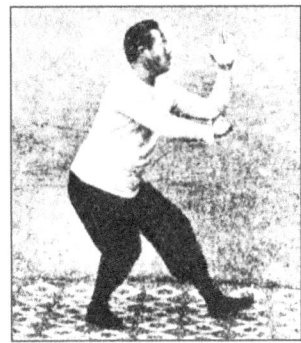 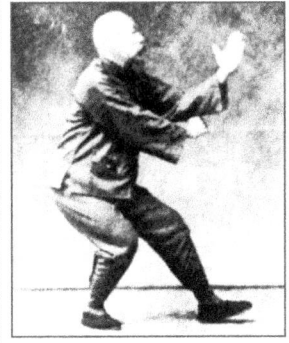

In fist under elbow, Master Yang (ca. 1918) and Chen Weiming (1932) reflect long, low postures. Yang's head is awry and neither is erect nor as relaxed as he could have been.

Some of these postures may not be stiff—though they appear to be so—but they are not quite accurate. Zheng Manqing stressed accuracy. Ben Lo, who was Zheng's first student in Taiwan, has said he was taught privately, posture by posture. That is, Zheng would not teach him a new posture until he had the current one down pat. As part of this training, Zheng taught that the postures had to be done both outwardly and inwardly yin. This confirmed the *Classics* and concealed the function of the form.

This may explain, at least partly, the seeming inaccuracy of some of the Yang/Chen photos. (Though the book was published in 1925, the photos may have been taken as much as a decade earlier.) In other words, they may have posed in the yang aspect, showing function, while Zheng's yin forms deliberately obscured this use. Either that, or they tried to pose the postures just as they did them daily—that is, with more of a yin emphasis—but were then made self-conscious by the camera.

By the time of the photo session for Master Yang's 1934 book (Yang, 1934), his form looks much better (or at least more like we do it now). Yang himself admitted his form had improved much in the interim, despite the fact that he had gained ninety pounds. However, the added bulk cost Yang some flexibility, notably on bow postures, in which he is unable to turn his rear foot inward from ninety degrees. While Yang was just too obese to make it, one wonders if this impediment has led many Yang-style teachers unknowingly to teach the bow posture without the turn-in to this day (Yang, 1983; Dong, 1948, 1953).[10]

Where We Come Out

Later in the thirties, Master Yang died (1936), Japan invaded (1937), and the Chinese government retreated westward to Chongqing in Sichuan Province.

After the Japanese surrender, Professor Zheng returned to Shanghai from Sichuan and met up with his old friend Chen Weiming, who had also survived the war. Zheng showed Chen the manuscript of his *Thirteen Chapters*, which he had written during the war. Chen was pleased with it, writing in his preface to the published work that it was excellent, kept strictly to Master Yang's original principles, and gave students a fine path to follow. In every respect, he wrote, it accorded with his own *Questions and Answers on Taijiquan*, written in 1929.

In the same preface, Chen stated that Master Yang had given Zheng Manqing all the secret oral transmissions, and that "no one else had ever heard them." He also mentioned that, in Sichuan, Zheng had met "an extraordinary man, studied with him, and made great progress" (Wile, 1985: 1–2).

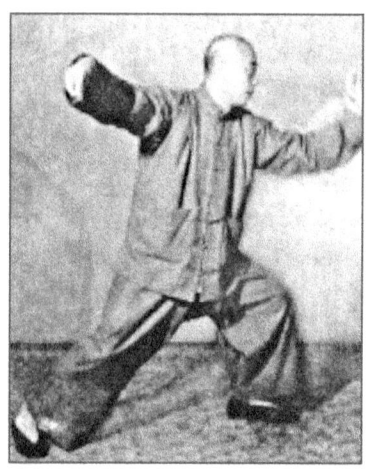

Dong Yingjie in single whip.

From the evidence, we know Chen Weiming was exceptional in both the theory and practice of taiji. We've seen his appreciation for the real taiji versus the normal taiji (which is to say the abnormal), and we've seen how he impressed his students. For example, the popular writer Xiang Kairan (Hsiang K'ai-jan), who often used martial art themes in his fiction, recalled Chen's pushhands skill during the twenties in Shanghai. Xiang, who had pushed with such adepts as Master Yang, Xu Yusheng, and Liu Ennuan, wrote of Chen Weiming that, like Master Yang, he liked ward-off and press but didn't use power. Instead, he "merely insinuated me lightly into a position from which I could neither dodge nor neutralize" (Hsiang, 1987).

Notwithstanding Chen's great abilities, he lacked one thing. Professor Zheng, honest almost to a fault, disclosed it in his *Manran san lun* [*Three treatises of Man-*

ran], published in Taibei in 1974. In the context of using *jin* (intrinsic energy) from the sinews instead of *li* (strength) from the bones, the Professor wrote, "My classmate Chen Weiming studied taiji for several decades, but when it came to the difference between strength and intrinsic energy, he was not able to get to the bottom of it" (Wile, 1985: 148).

Some may think Zheng's words gratuitous, particularly about such a close friend as Chen. I think he wrote them, however, because principle and truth precede conventional courtesies. The principle of resilient intrinsic energy was so important as to demand it. After all, if his dear friend, Chen Weiming, one of the finest boxers in China, failed to fully understand the difference, then it must be doubly hard for the rest of us.

The idea of intrinsic energy from the sinews is not hard to understand intellectually, but to practice it and express it with your body, that is a far different thing. Zheng Manqing was not gloating over the shortfall of his old friend so much as commiserating over the struggle. Two friends had sought the knowledge, but only one had achieved it.

Acknowledgements

Thanks go to several persons who helped with this article. Warren Conner, Barbara Davis, Russ Mason, and Joe Svinth reviewed the text, Dan and Harry Johnston aided on graphics, and Ben Lo provided much substance. Barbara Davis translated parts of Chen Weiming's works (1925, 1927) that appear with my modifications in this article.

Notes

1. Although more sustained in Shanghai, studio teaching had occurred somewhat earlier in Beijing. The man spearheading it there was Xu Yusheng (1879–1945). A student of Yang Jianhou, Song Shuming, and other greats, Xu was an intellectual greatly respected in Beijing. In 1912 he became vice-director of the Beijing Physical Education Research Association, teaching mainly taiji. In this venue, he was able to invite famed colleagues such as Yang Shaohou, Liu Caijen, Yang Shao, and Wu Jianquan to teach taiji there at least occasionally. In 1921 Xu published a book called *Diagrammatic Explanations of the Taijiquan Postures* [*Taijiquan shi tujie*]. We can see him in photographs in Chen Weiming's *The Art of Taijiquan* (Chen, 1925: 48, 50).

2   Also in 1928, Wu Jianquan moved with his family from Beijing to Shanghai, where he taught his idiosyncratic Wu style, further establishing Shanghai as a center for taiji. Wu's father, Wu Quanyu, had been a direct student of the famed Yang Banhou (Zee, 1992: 15).

3   Besides Shanghai, Yang also spent periods teaching in Nanjing, Hangzhou, Hankou, and Guangzhou. On these trips, he took along as assistants such men as Wu Huiquan, a 250-pound ex-wrestler, Dong Yingjie, Yang Kairu, Zhang Qinlin, and Fu Zhongwen.

4   When young, Shaohou had been given to his somewhat irascible uncle Banhou as a foster son and acquired some of that man's fiery temperament. This fieriness was reflected in Shaohou's teaching, which many regarded as so harsh that he couldn't keep students. Elsewhere, I've told of Shaohou's suicide in 1929 (Draeger & Smith, 1980: 39). Sources in Taiwan told me he took his life by nailing scissors to a table and then impaling his throat on them. The reason was that one of his students, a high government official, had left him for another teacher. (Doubtless Shaohou's harshness played a part in this departure.) Since then I've heard a less credible story in which Shaohou, while fencing with his beloved daughter, ran her through. This caused him such grief that he exited with the scissors. As I said, I prefer the more quotidian version to the sensational one and only mention it here to quash the latter with skepticism.

5   Although the story of Zhang Sanfeng as the creator of taiji has little historic weight, both Chen Weiming and Zheng Manqing openly subscribed to it, perhaps in deference to Yang family belief. If so, this seems too much of a kowtow.

6   "T'was ever thus," sayeth the Bard. More frictions and fights were (and are) caused by gossiping students than directly by teachers.

7   If true, it seems significant that Luchan hadn't even bothered to attend the match. This may speak more loudly than the match itself.

8   A longer set of 118 photographs done by Chen is appended at the back of the book. Since he has aged appreciably in these pictures, this set may not have been a part of the 1925 first edition, but added in a later edition.

9   Similarly, as far as I know, there were no films made of Vaslav Nijinsky, the greatest dancer of all time. All we have of this artist, who could fly onto the stage through a window, leap head down with his feet straight up, and soar and hover before descending, are descriptions, posed photographs, and legends. "I am God in the body; everybody has this feeling. Only nobody uses it; I do use it," Nijinsky wrote before dancing his last dance in 1919 and going mad at the age of twenty-nine (Hallander, 1996: 9). I do not mean to compare Nijinsky with Yang, but say only that still photographs are inadequate for capturing the movement, look, or essence of either man.

[10] Yang Zhenduo turns in slightly on bow posture, as does Dong Yingjie. However, neither man turns his foot to forty-five, as Zheng taught (Yang, 1983; Dong, 1948, 1953).

[11] Wang Yannian and several other leading lights in Taiwan told me that, excluding Zhang Qinlin and Zheng Manqing, the most skilled of Master Yang's seniors was Chen Weiming. In 1973 Zheng, a man not given to lavish praise, told the New York City class that his elder brother under Master Yang, Li Yaxuan, had extraordinary skill unapproached on the mainland. Ben Lo remembers Zheng speaking glowingly of Li and rating Li's skills higher than Zheng's own.

Romanization		
Pinyin	Wade-Giles	Chinese
bagua	pakua	八卦
Beijing	Peiching	北京
Chenjiagou	Ch'en chia kou	陳家溝
Chen Zhangxing	Ch'en Chang-hsing	陳長興
Chen Weiming	Ch'en Wei-ming	陳微明
Dong Yingjie	Tung Ying-chieh	董英傑
feiteng	fei t'eng	飛騰
Fu Zhongwen	Fu Chung-wen	傅鍾文
Guangzhou	Gaung-chou	廣州
Henan	Honan	河南
li	li	力
Li Yaxuan	Li Ya-hsuan	李雅軒
qigong	ch'i kung	氣功
Sichuan	Szechuan	四川
Sun Lutang	Sun Lu-t'ang	孫祿堂
Wang Lanting	Wang Lan-t'ing	王蘭亭
Wu Huichuan	Wu Hui-ch'uan	武匯川
Wu Jianquan	Wu Chien-ch'üan	吳鑑泉
Wu Quanyou	Wu Ch'uan-yu	吳全佑
xingyi	hsing-i	形意
Yang Banhou	Yang Pan-hou	楊班侯
Yang Chengfu	Yang Ch'eng-fu	楊澄甫
Yang Jianhou	Yang Chien-hou	楊健侯
Yang Luchan	Yang Lu-ch'an	楊露禅
Yang Shaohou	Yang Shao-hou	楊少侯
Yang Zhenduo	Yang Chen-tuo	楊振鐸
Zheng Manqing	Cheng Man-ch'ing	鄭曼青
Zhang Qinlin	Chang Ch'in-lin	張欽霖
Zhang Sanfeng	Chang San-feng	張三丰

Bibliography

Chen, W. (1927). *Taiji jian* [Taiji sword]. Shanghai: Self-published.

Chen, W. (1925). *Taijiquan shu* [Art of taiji boxing]. Shanghai: Self-published.

Dong, Y. (1948, 1953). *Taijiquan shi-yi* [An explanation of taiji boxing]. Hong Kong: Commercial Press.

Draeger, D., & Smith, R. (1980). *Comprehensive Asian fighting arts*. Tokyo: Kodansha.

Hallander, A. (25 Jan., 1996). God in the body. *London review of books*, 18 (2): 9–10.

Hsiang, K. (Sept.–Oct., 1987). Push-hands. (K. Cohen, Trans.). *Bubbling well journal*.

Wile, D. (1985). *Cheng Man-ch'ing's advanced t'ai-chi form instructions*. Brooklyn: Sweet Ch'i Press.

Xu, Y. (1921). *Taijiquan shi tujie* [A diagrammatic explanation of the taijiquan postures]. Shanghai: Self-published.

Yang, C. (1934). *Taijiquan ti yong quan shu* [Complete principles and function of taijiquan]. Shanghai: Self-published.

Yang, Z. (1983). *Yang style taijiquan*. Hong Kong: Hai Feng Publishing Co.

Zee, W. (April, 1992). Wu Ying-hua on Wu style. *T'ai chi*. Los Angeles: Wayfarer Publications.

Zheng, M. (1974). *Manran san lun* [Three treatises of Manran]. Taibei: Zhonghua shuju.

Dalü and Some Tigers
by Robert W. Smith, M.A.

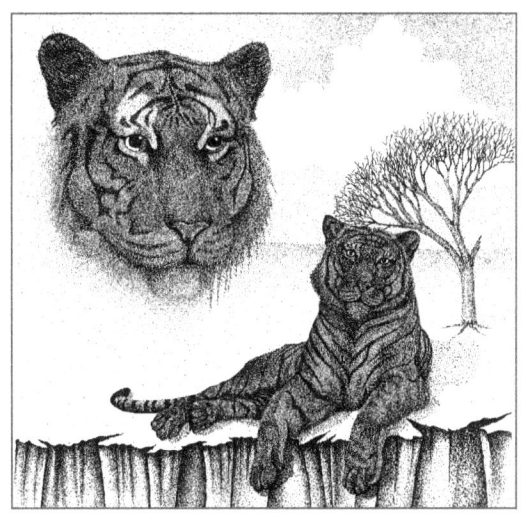

Illustration by Gene Scott.
All photographs courtesy of Robert W. Smith

Introduction

Other than weapons play, taiji comprises four categories:
- **Basic Solo Form** (*gongjia*, literally "task framework")—having twenty-four, thirty-seven, 108, 128, 150, or more individual postures, depending on the system.
- **Push-Hands** (*tuishou*)—done with a partner in either a fixed- or free-step atmosphere, featuring ward-off, rollback, press, and push; oriented largely to the cardinal directions.
- **Large Rollback** (*dalü*)—a set routine with a partner, emphasizing the use of pull (*cai*), split (*lieh*), shoulder strike (*gao*), and elbow strike (*chou*); oriented to the four corners or diagonals.
- **Dispersing Hands** (*sanshou*)—a mock fighting set with a partner in which both use a prearranged series of hand and foot techniques for attacking and defending.

Of these, only the form, the crucible of the art, is done slowly and by oneself. The rest are practiced at a normal or appropriate speed in pairs. The form requires slowness and evenness.[1]

Here I want to dilate on dalü, the shortest of the set exercises. The name is one of those special terms that crept into the taiji patois at an early date. It does not translate very well.[2] Some call it push-hands of the four corners. Close maybe, but not close enough. Sensing hands, which I prefer to push-hands, is a fairly free practice and softly (a word that needs shouting, not murmuring) competitive. It is a disciplined balance, in fact, of the competitive and the cooperative. However, while the play in dalü involves two people, one competes only with oneself. In cooperating and moving in accord with the *Taiji Classics*, both players gain immeasurably.

While Professor Zheng Manqing devoted a few pages to dalü in his seminal *Thirteen Chapters* (1950), he used only five photographs to illustrate the concept (he posed with Li Shoujian).[3] For our book, *T'ai-chi: The "Supreme Ultimate" Exercise for Health, Sport, and Self-Defense* (1967), Professor Zheng provided text and photos done with Liang Tongcai. Because of space constraints, these dalü photos and text were never used. I have incorporated them here. The basic set is done here by Benjamin Lo and myself.[4]

Directions and Explanations of Photographs

Directions correspond to Mr. Lo's movements.
The attacker and defender swap roles in photo 11.

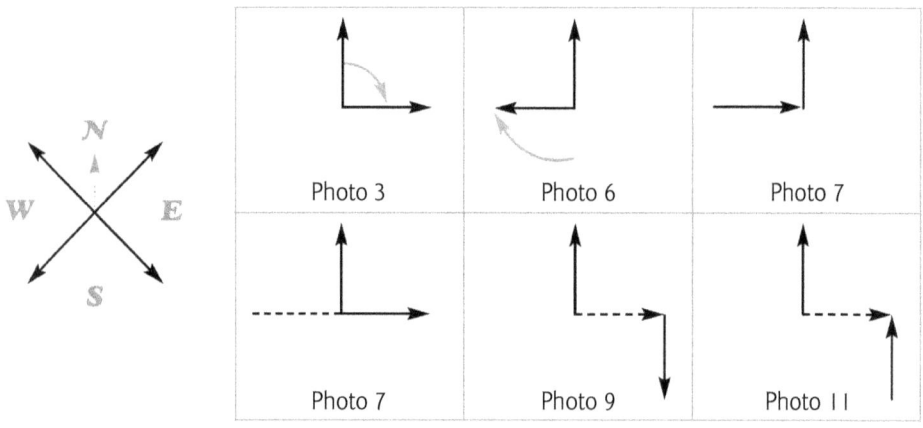

About Dalü

Dalü is usually done at normal speed, but for variety it can be done slow or fast. You and your partner start with your right hands joined, and later round the set out by starting with your left hands joined.

As in push-hands, quantity is less important than quality. Stand upright and relaxed. Though rooted, move lightly with celerity in absorbing, sticking, neutralizing, and countering. Be soft and pliable. No resistance and no letting go. Yield a little and then turn. Breathe naturally through your nose. Most importantly: keep your mind at your navel. The techniques used during dalü include pull (cai), split (lieh), elbow strike (chou), and shoulder strike (gao). These four were part of the original taiji set of thirteen postures and supplement the four basic techniques of push-hands, namely ward-off (*peng*), rollback (*lu*), press (*ji*), and push (*an*). The remaining five techniques of the original thirteen are associated mainly with "dispersing hands" (sanshou), and have to do with the "attitudes" of advancing, retreating, looking left and right, and maintaining one's center.

Doing Dalü

Smith and Lo face each other on the cardinal direction (photo 1). Next they ward off with their right wrists, the hands forming press (photo 2). Each shifts his weight to his left foot, leaving his right foot empty. (This is the conventional beginning. In real use, Smith has struck at Lo, who blocks the attack with ward-off.) Now Smith shifts his weight to his right foot and steps forward with his left while Lo shifts his weight to his right foot and pivots on his left to the right (photo 3). In photo 4 Professor Zheng, right, and Liang Tongcai show Zheng's press unfolding so that his left hand is on Liang's forearm to prevent him from using his elbow strike. In photo 5 Zheng pivots on his left foot while Liang steps forward with his left.

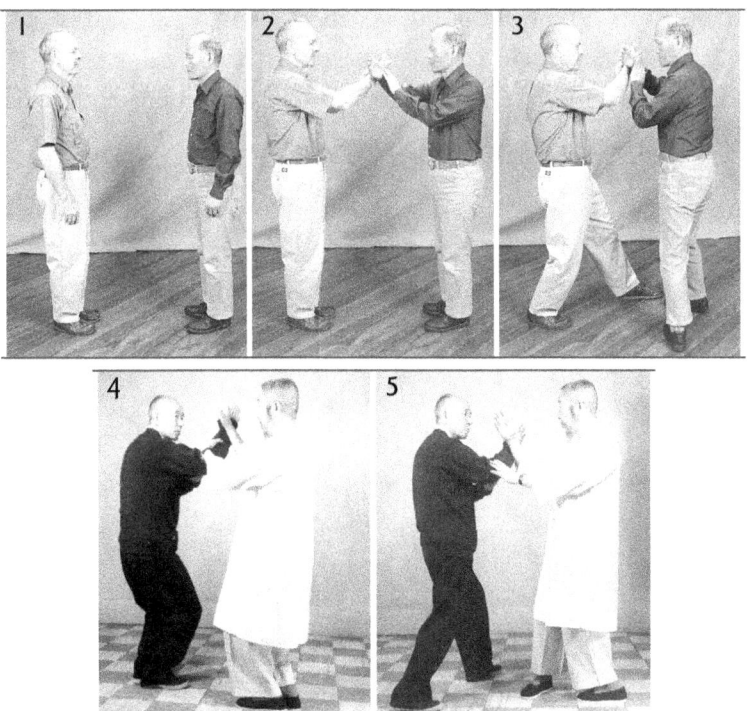

Smith next steps forward with his right foot near Lo's groin, causing Lo to circle his right leg to the rear right corner. Rolling back with his left elbow on Smith's right elbow while pulling Smith's right wrist with the thumb and middle finger of his right hand (photo 6a; 6b is a rear view of the same action).

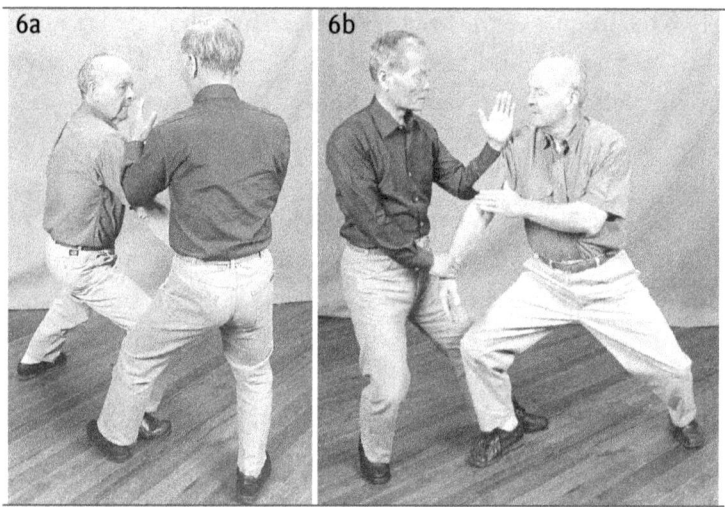

Next, when Smith neutralizes Lo's pull, Lo circles his right hand rearward and counterclockwise, then back to the front in an attempt to slap Smith's face with his right palm (split) while simultaneously stepping forward with his right foot. As Lo steps forward with split, Smith steps backward with his right foot, bringing his feet together, and warding off Lo's split (photo 7a; 7b is a reverse shot).

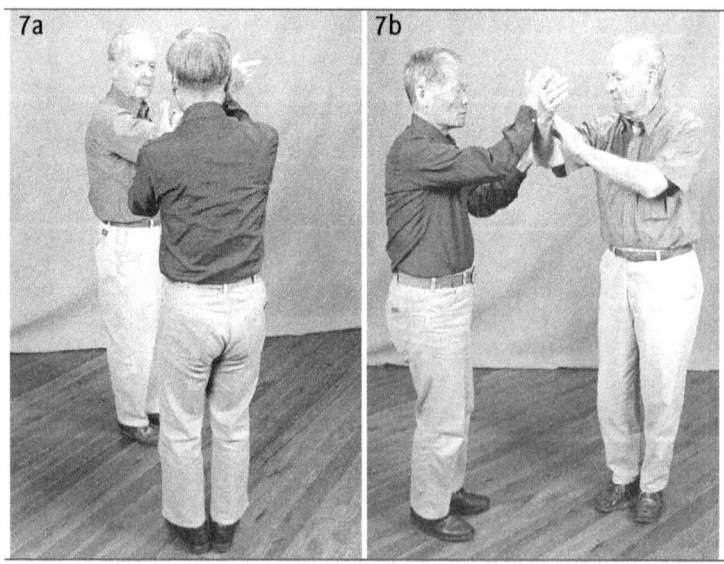

Next, Smith toes his left foot inward and begins to withdraw his right foot to the rear (photo 8) while clasping Lo's right wrist lightly with the thumb and middle finger and pulling him forward using his left elbow on Lo's right elbow in rollback. While this is occurring, Lo is stepping with his left foot and then placing his right foot forward, near Smith's groin, using shoulder strike (photo 9a). Although oriented to a different corner, I have juxtaposed Liang's rollback opposing Zheng's shoulder strike to show Liang's vertical left arm here (photo 9b). In photo 9c, a reverse shot of photo 9a, Smith has neutralized Lo's shoulder strike and is folding down from rollback.

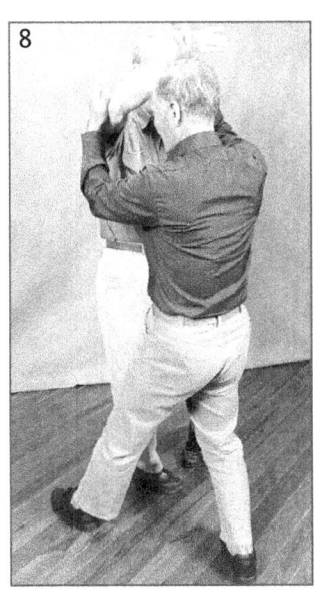

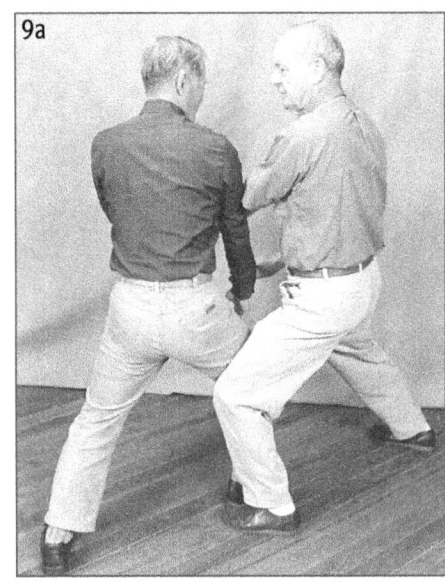

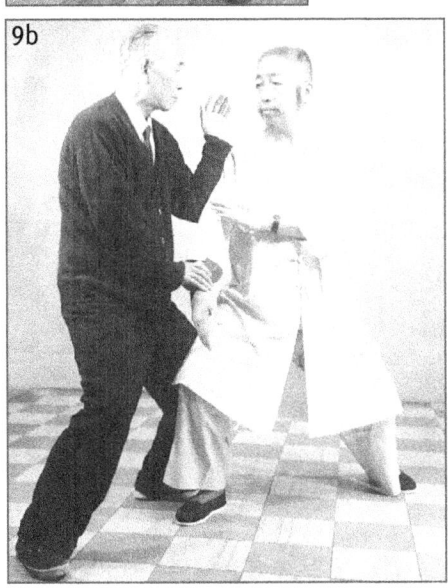

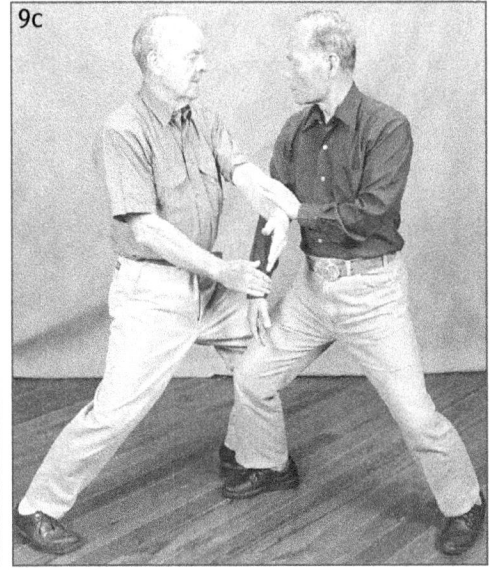

Resuming the proper orientation, Smith takes his right arm back, circling it counterclockwise to the front, attempting to slap (split) Lo's face. Smith's right foot accompanies his strike with a right ward-off while stepping back with his right foot to join his left (photo 10; photo 11 shows this posture frozen for function with Zheng in Lo's role and Liang in Smith's, but oriented toward a different corner).

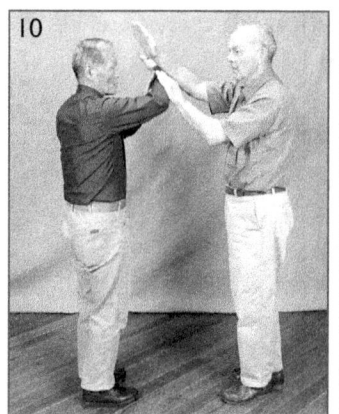 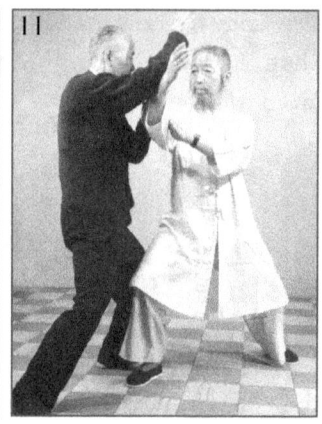

In photo 12 Smith steps forward with his left foot and then with his right near Lo's groin. Lo uses rollback, pulling Smith's right wrist lightly with his right thumb and middle finger, and putting his left elbow on Smith's right elbow. This neutralizes Smith's shoulder strike. Lo then withdraws his right hand (photo 13). Now, with Zheng in Lo's role and Liang in Smith's in the correct orientation, Zheng circles his right hand counterclockwise to the rear and then to the front in split, striking Liang's face (photo 14). (Note that their splits, Liang's in photo 11 and Zheng's in photo 14, are frozen to show use, while in the splits done by Lo and Smith, the legs accompany the strike to show form.)

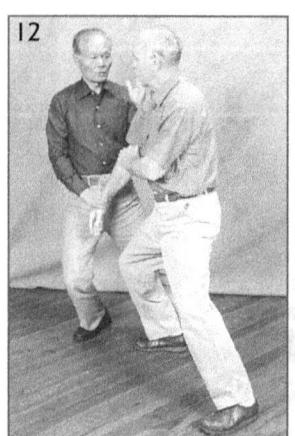 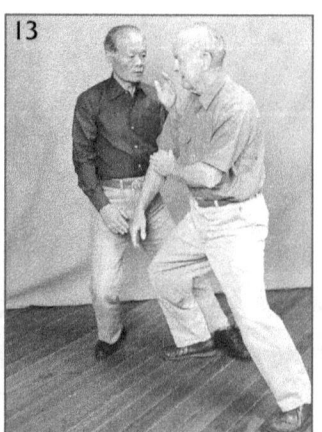 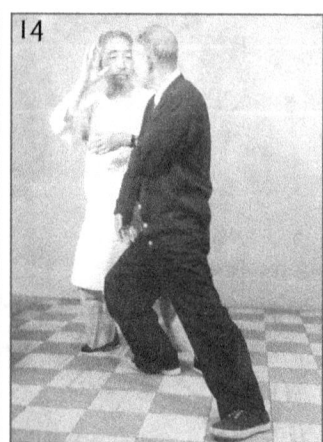

Concluding, as Lo splits, stepping forward with his right foot to join his left, Smith steps back with his right foot to join his left while intercepting Lo's right slap with right ward-off (photo 15).

Confucius once said, "If I give you one corner [of a square of a handkerchief, for example], and you cannot find the other three corners for yourself, am I obliged to find them for you?" Here, I have given you dalü done to three of the four corners. You can find the last yourself. And finding, do. And doing, learn. And learning, enjoy.

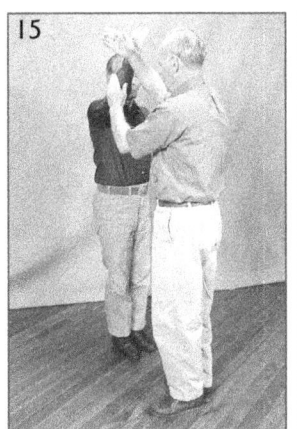
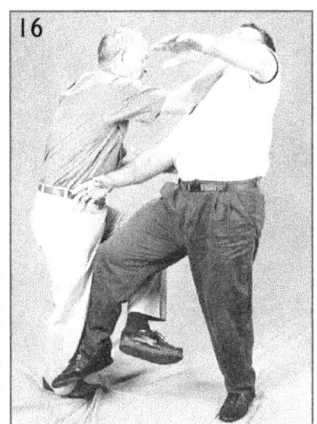

The Uses of Dalü

Like the solo form, dalü is awash with function. In pull, you use the thumb and middle finger to hold your partner's wrist lightly and throw him out. In this regard, it is like brush knee, in which it is contained. In split, when he pushes my elbow, I yield, follow, and neutralize his strength by slapping his head with my palm. One can see this technique in the posture step back and ride the tiger. Elbow strike can be used in step forward, deflect downward, parry, and punch, at the outset of dalü following the initial joining of hands, and in many other postures. Shoulder strike follows lift hands, and is applicable whenever the opponent pulls on you.

I mentioned above that split is similar to step back and ride the tiger. In the latter, however, your left foot is empty, whereas in split it can be full, depending on the circumstances. If empty, your left foot can be used to sweep your opponent's approaching foot in concert with your split (photo 16, step back and ride the tiger).

Another tiger posture is embrace tiger and return to mountain. Zheng's short form has three tiger postures that can be used against someone whose split or punch has miscarried. In photos 17 and 18 Zheng ducks Liang's strike, wraps his right arm around Liang's back, and grabs his right knee. He then stands up and upends Liang by pulling sharply upward with both hands to the left.

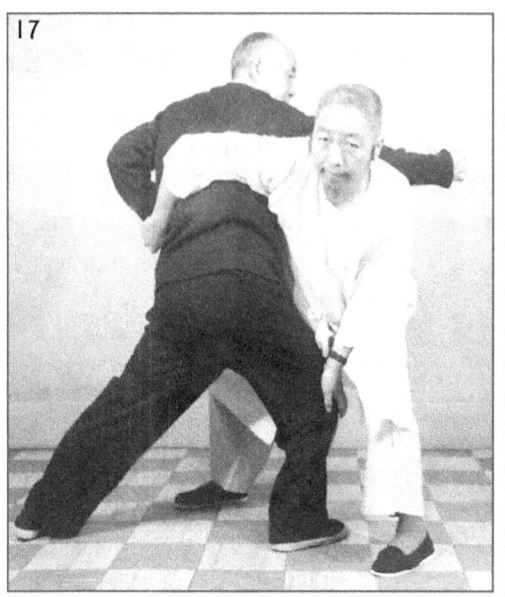 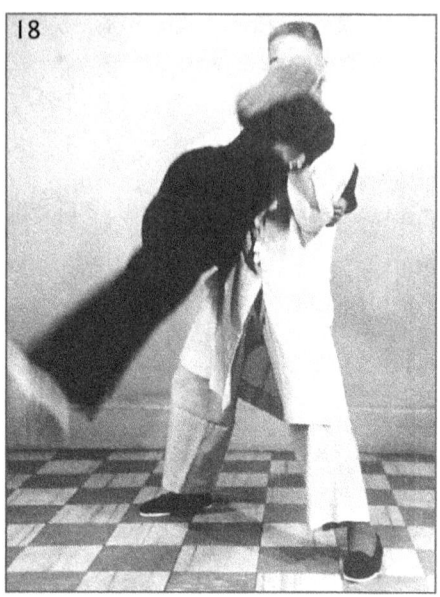

Function of embrace tiger and return to mountain
(Professor Zheng and Liang Tongcai).

Speaking of tigers,
let me tell you of one.
It was a special tiger—
the only one Zheng ever met.

• • •

Zheng Meets a Tiger

In an introduction to the translation of *Cheng Tzu's Thirteen Treatises on T'ai-chi Ch'uan* (1985: 13–15), Min Xiaoqi (Min Hsiao-chi), a celebrated authority on Chinese literature, stated that he met three extraordinary men in his lifetime. One was an eighty-year-old monk with a child's face who gathered rare herbs in the mountains of Zhejiang Province by climbing and jumping through pines and vines like a monkey. Later, Min met and was awed by a seventy-year-old Daoist priest with a young appearance and a resonant voice who had meditated for forty years. Zheng Manqing was the third outstanding man he met. In enumerating Zheng's excellences, which included medicine, painting, calligraphy, and taiji, Min mentioned that Zheng liked to climb mountains that had deep gorges. "Danger did not deter him," Min wrote. "Once he met a tiger but was not frightened because he was internally strong and his mind was calm" (Lo & Inn, 1985: 12).[5]

Professor Zheng told Tam Gibbs of his encounter with the tiger, and Tam recounted it to me years ago. Zheng was walking on a meandering path up a mountain, probably in Zhejiang, when he met a tiger coming down. Because the path was narrow, there was no way for the two to pass without incident. So when Zheng saw the huge animal coming around a turn toward him, he slowly retreated to the outside of the path until he came to the edge of the cliff overlooking the gorge below. Just as he noticed his plight, his hand touched a sapling growing from the cliff edge. Keeping his eyes steadily on the tiger, Zheng pulled and bent the pliable sapling back for its full length, ten feet or so, and held the leafed top in the face of the tiger in the taiji movement step back and repulse the monkey (photo 20). Note well: he did not shake the tree to scare the tiger. A tiger is unlikely to be frightened by either a man or a small tree, but he may become excited by a tree brandished in his face. No, Zheng merely put it near the tiger's nose and held it there. After a time, the tiger broke off his baleful look into Zheng's eyes, shook his head slightly, and sauntered on past Zheng down the mountain path. Zheng stood up and released the tree, and in a rush, the cool, imperturbable face he had shown the tiger disappeared and his whole body shook uncontrollably. After a while, the shakes subsided and, with an occasional look over his shoulder, he continued up the path.

Some readers will not believe this story, a quite understandable reaction given the state of truth in media. However, I think it probably happened. For starters, Professor Zheng was not given to "terminological inexactitudes," as Winston Churchill called lies. He was no politician. He would sometimes forget details, but deceit was alien to his nature. Nor did he make himself a hero by bare-handedly killing the tiger as the Tiger Swami in P. Yogananda's *The Autobiography of a Yogi* (1948: 67–68) reportedly did. Professor Zheng was no hero, merely a survivor. Given the tightness of the passage and the fact that Chinese tigers are presumably as hungry as Chinese people, it was a close thing. Perhaps the tiger had eaten recently and when he met no antagonism from the small man he chanced upon, with only a focused desire to be left alone, the tiger gave him his space. Instinctively, Zheng made the right choice. If he had panicked, the animal would have picked up on his fear; if he had shaken the sapling aggressively, the tiger probably would have mauled him grievously.

Curiously, in Taiwan many years before I heard this story from Tam Gibbs, Zheng and I had been discussing function and he spoke of the ferocity of a tiger as being short lived. If one could survive the first charge, he said (and his "if" was a beaut), one might have a chance to escape. The tiger does not economize; his attack is total, and thus he tires quickly. Biologists agree on this. Like all cats, the tiger cannot maintain exertion for long because of its narrow chest and relatively small lungs. Did Zheng's focused mind have room for this contingency? I doubt it.

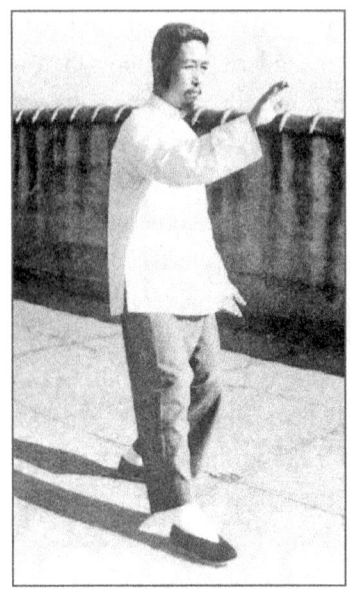 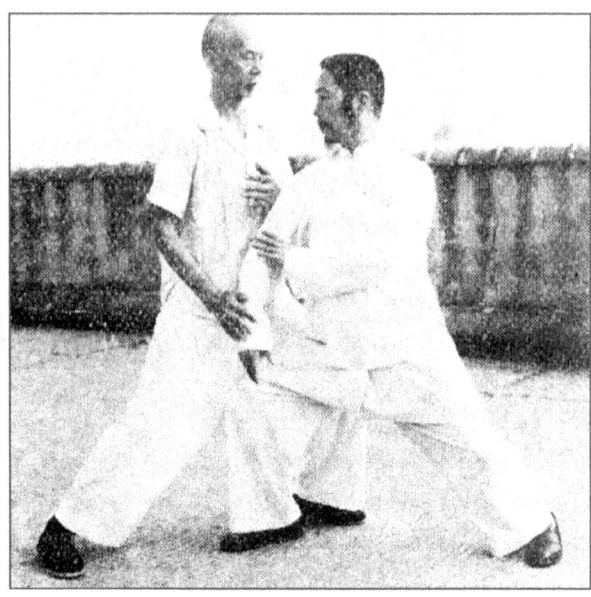

Zheng in repulse monkey and with Li Shoujian doing dalü.

So much for the tiger. During his exposition of his three great men, Mr. Min ranked Zheng Manqing above the other two by saying Zheng "was a great man compared with those who stayed in old temples and remote mountains, who preferred to seek quietness and protect themselves rather than participate in the country's destiny or the rise and fall of the world" (Lo & Inn, 1985: 15). Mr. Min makes an insightful point. Perhaps Professor Zheng's greatest gift was that in an always eventful, sometimes tumultuous life, he remained rooted and relaxed while living and raising a family in the real world. In letting the world go past instead of through him, he minded his center and never left off meditating. And according to the ancients, this moving meditation is superior to the static meditation done in monasteries.

Notes

[1] Yang Shouting reportedly had a "small frame" taiji set he taught privately comprising seventy-three postures (two hundred, counting repetitions) that was done in two to three minutes (Lim, n.d.: 36). If true, this was racing with a vengeance. In the black and white film we made of Zheng in Taibei in 1960, he did the thirty-seven postures (sixty-five, counting repetitions) in about three

minutes. Though impatient that morning and running late, he still did it correctly, separating all the way. Hurried, his form still effused beauty. However, Mr. Lim would double the number of postures and triple the total with repetitions. I do not think it could be done and still fall under the rubric of taiji, as such speed defies, if it does not defile, the *Classics*, where Li Yiyu writes, "In practicing the form we want slowness not speed"; and Wu Yuxiang advises that one should "outwardly exhibit calmness and peace" (Lo, 1979: 47, 82). Physiologically, taiji works by relaxing the cerebrum. Without slowness, this will not happen (*China Sports*, 1980: 7–8). Mr. Lim is stingy on sources. Here is one to confound him. Yang Chengfu's nephew (and a famed taiji adept in his own right), Fu Zhongwen, said in an interview a few years back, "There is none nor was there ever a fast set in the Yang style traditional system. People who practice a fast set and call it the Yang style are not practicing the traditional Yang style taijiquan. Any fast set was developed by students of the Yang style. The form takes normally twenty to thirty minutes to practice, and it is practiced in a slow, evenly paced manner" (Yu & Sharp, 1993). Even Dong Yingjie, a senior under Master Yang, often practiced an auxiliary short "flying form." The late Kuo Lienying showed me his normal-speed "Guangping" form, said to be derived from Yang Banhou, in Taibei in 1962. However, there was little separation of weight evident. Some other schools do taiji at normal speed, a prime example being Sun Lutang's *houbu jia*, or "lively pace form." Other schools, such as the Chenjiagou style, sporadically exceed even normal speed, or create a variant fast form as a break from the ennui of doing it slowly. However, none of the fast forms I have seen separates the weight into one leg as required by the *Classics*. There is no great harm in these quickie steps, as long as they do not distract from or become confused with real taiji.

2 As Bix Beiderbeck, our finest jazz cornetist, said of the prose of the noted French novelist Marcel Proust.

3 Though I cannot recall meeting Li Shoujian during my stay in Taiwan (1959–1962), I heard about him. One Chinese friend told me that he had seen Li do taiji on the lawn on a windless day and his indescribably beautiful postures made the grass move.

4 Ben Lo was Professor Zheng's first student when Zheng relocated to Taiwan from the mainland in 1949. I met Laoshi ("teacher") a decade later, and both Lo and I are still trying to decipher and live life by practicing taiji (it is difficult, but it beats working). Modest to a fault, Lo has forgotten, if you will forgive the cliché, more taiji than most so-called masters know. We are old friends, having been born within four months of each other in 1926–27, and I bow deeply to him for his help with this article.

5 In his translation (1982), Douglas Wile has Min, whose given name he misspells as Hsia-chi, say that Zheng "often encountered tigers." If Zheng had met tigers often, we would never have heard of him . . .

Bibliography

China Sports Series. (1980). *Simplified taijiquan*. Beijing: China Sports Series 1.

Lim, T. (n.d.). *The origins and history of taijiquan*. Singapore: n.p.

Lo, B., et al. (1979). *The essence of t'ai chi ch'uan*. Richmond, CA: North Atlantic Books.

Lo, P., & Inn, M. (1985). *Cheng Tzu's thirteen treatises on tai-chi ch'uan*. Berkeley, CA: North Atlantic Books.

Wile, D. (Trans.). (1982). *Master Cheng's thirteen chapters on t'ai-chi ch'uan*. Brooklyn, NY: Sweet Ch'i Press.

Yu, W., & Sharp, G. (April 1993). Fu Zhong Wen: A family legend. *Inside kung-fu*, pp. 44–46.

Yogananda, P. (1946). *The autobiography of a yogi*. New York: The Philosophical Library.

Zheng, M. (1950). *Zhengzi taijiquan shisan pian* [Master Zheng's thirteen treatises on taijiquan]. Sections 1 and 2. Taibei: n.p.

Zheng, M., & Smith, R. (1967). *T'ai-chi: The "supreme ultimate" exercise for health, sport, and self-defense*. Rutland, VT: Charles E. Tuttle, Co.

Liu Xiheng: Memories of a Taiji Sage

by Benjamin Lo, Xu Yizhong, Yuan Weiming,
Xu Zhengmei, and Danny Emerick[1]
Compiled by Russ Mason, M.A.

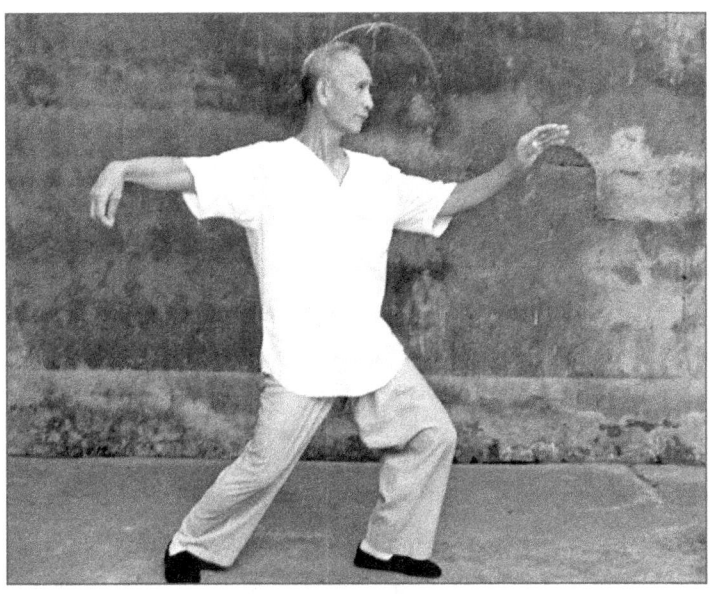

Liu demonstrates the single-whip posture.
Photo courtesy of Yuan Weiming.

General Introduction

Liu Xiheng's master, the late Professor Zheng Manqing, was a close disciple of Yang Chengfu in the 1930s[2] and was the scribe of Yang's 1934 book, *Essence and Applications of Taijiquan*.[3] Zheng is well known in America as a paragon of traditional Chinese arts and culture and, in particular, as the originator of the thirty-seven-posture short form of Yang-style taijiquan, which became popular here in the early 1960s and is still widely practiced. From the time of his arrival in the US until his passing in 1975, Professor Zheng worked to preserve and research traditional Chinese arts and to teach and interpret these treasures for westerners. In addition to being noted for his soft and effective skill in taijiquan push-hands (tuishou) and the use of the double-edged sword (taiji jian), Professor Zheng is remembered for his deep commitment to the transmission of the classical principles of taiji and to the practice of taijiquan, not only as a martial art, but also as a Dao of living and personal cultivation.[4]

Liu Xiheng was a living embodiment of this Dao of taijiquan. Left in charge of Zheng's Taibei Shizhong Study Society while "the Professor" was teaching in America (establishing what was known in English as the New York Shr Jung School), Liu did his best to carry forward his master's mission. Later, at the time of Zheng's passing, Liu was officially installed as head of the Taibei school, and he continued to serve in this capacity as head disciple and "gatekeeper" of the Zheng tradition in Taiwan from 1975 until his retirement in 1986.[5] After retirement, Liu settled down to a quiet, contemplative life as a Buddhist layperson, pursuing the practice of meditation and teaching a small, dedicated group of Chinese and international taijiquan students who met for practice first at his home in Taibei and later in parks and various nearby venues.

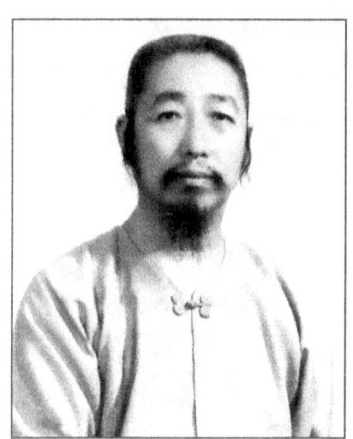
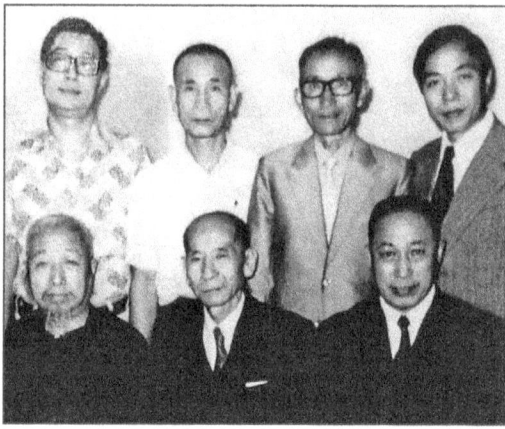

Left: Zheng Manqing. Right, first row, from left: Zheng Manqing, Mr. Hong (friend and legal advisor from Hong Kong), and Wang Yannian. Back row, from left: Mr. Yang (a lawyer friend), Liu Xiheng, Tao Bianxiang, and Xu Yizhong (current association president). Courtesy of Zheng Manqing Jinian Guan.

Although the field of martial arts is sometimes marred by ego and self-promotion, Liu worked quietly and modestly, honoring his master, nurturing students, and caring nothing for the limelight. A shining example of traditional *wude* (martial virtues or morality), Liu's humble character, diligence, and unimpeachable integrity were an inspiration to all who had the privilege of knowing him. In regard to martial applications, Liu's neutralizing and discharging skills in tuishou were marvelous to experience. Those who were fortunate enough to cross arms with Liu and to feel his gentle touch often came away shaking their heads in amazement over the apparently effortless ease with which he was able to neutralize and send attackers flying away.

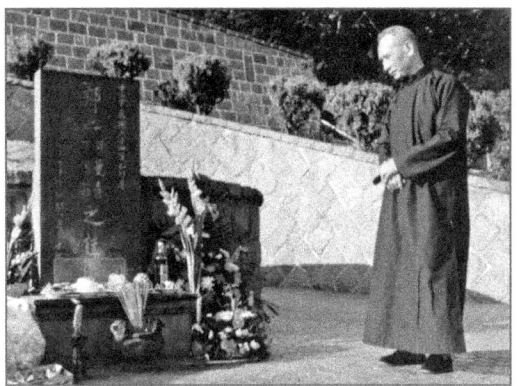 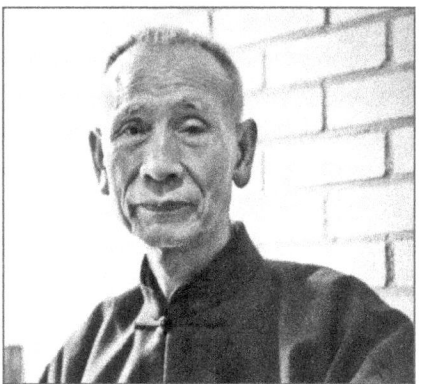

Liu pays his respects at Master Zheng's tomb;
Liu close-up. Photos courtesy of Yuan Weiming.

Liu often said softly and smilingly, "You must relax and eradicate every thought of using force. If you are not relaxed, you are crooked. If you are crooked, you are using force." And again, with twinkling eyes he urged, "We must learn to be tender, soft, and peaceful." Liu seasoned his conversation with frequent quotes from the Classics and from Professor Zheng: "The most important factors in taiji are honesty and sincerity, for without these qualities one can't advance."[6] Liu held that the essential thing was to apply the principles of taiji in daily life, to nurture character, and to grow as human beings in our care for others. For those who followed him, he was a living example of the Dao of taiji.

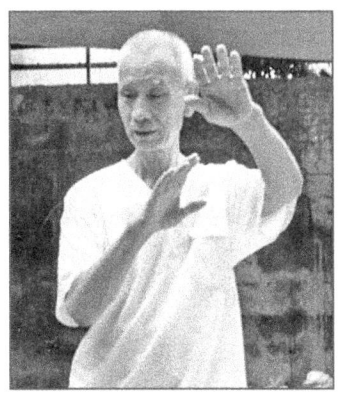 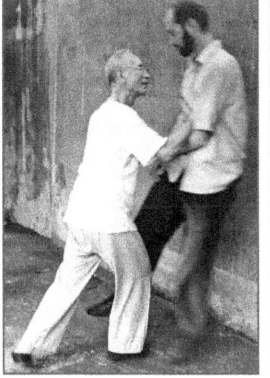 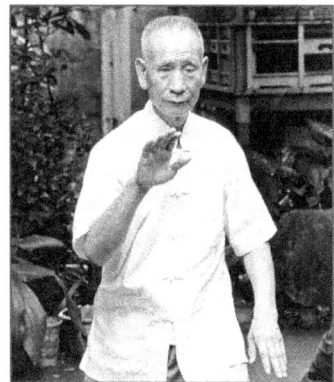

In the courtyard of his Taibei home,
Liu demonstrates fair lady works at shuttles (left),
brush knee (right), and uproots his student, Bill Tucker.
Photos courtesy of Yuan Weiming.

Notes

1. The first author is commonly known as Ben Lo or as Benjamin Pangjeng Lo. Because the pinyin romanization Luo Bangzhen is unfamiliar to the English-language audience, his pinyin romanization will not be used in this article, except for reference in the glossary. Likewise, the third author became known as "Yuan" Weiming due to a documentation error in the 1970s, when he came to the US for graduate studies. Pinyin spelling of his family name is "Ruan" and is given for reference in the glossary.
2. A number of Professor Zheng's books and articles have been translated into English and much has been written about him. For more background information and for extensive bibliographies of relevant texts, see numerous *Journal of Asian Martial Arts* back issues (e.g., Davis, 1996; Davis & Mann, 1996; Mason, 2008; Mason, 2001; Smith, 1997; Smith, 1995, etc.), as well as books (e.g., Cheng & Smith, 1967; Cheng, 1950/1985; Lowenthal, 1991; Smith, 1974; Smith, 1999; Wile, 2007, etc.).
3. See Louis Swaim's English translation of Yang's masterwork (Yang, 1934/2005). See also details of Zheng's collaborative role as Yang's disciple and scribe (e.g., Mason, 2008: 36; Mason, 2006: 92; Yang, 1988; Yang, 1993; Yang, 1934/2005: xi; and Yu and Sharp, 1993: 44–46).
4. For an exposition of Zheng's quest for a "unified Dao," see Davis (1996).
5. The sources of this biographical information are the compiler's personal conversations with Liu Xiheng and his disciples, as well as the compiler's own research and study in Taibei during visits to Southeast Asia in 1989–1990, 1998, and 2006. Although disinclined to make public statements, Liu did publish one article in a Kaohsiung periodical and, from time to time, articles and comments were published about him. A few of his lectures have been transcribed. For a fine sample of Liu's own views on taijiquan, see Rick Halstead's English translation of Liu's article, "The concept of central equilibrium in t'ai chi ch'uan," in *T'ai Chi Player* (Liu, 1985) and reprinted in *Taijiquan Journal* (Liu, 1985/2002). For more background information on Liu, see the excellent articles by Lin Farley (1986) and Bill Tucker (2008).
6. See Robert W. Smith's description of Liu (Smith, 1999: 313–314). For more quotations from Liu, see Lin Farley (1986).

Introduction to Benjamin Lo's Memorial Article

Benjamin Lo (Luo Bangzhen) is a well-known proponent of taijiquan and has taught in the United States for many years.[7] He became Zheng Manqing's first taijiquan student in Taiwan soon after Zheng's emigration from the Chinese mainland in 1949. As a teenager, Lo suffered from a serious neurological disorder. After seeking Zheng's services as a doctor of traditional Chinese medicine, he began his study of taijiquan as a part of his treatment. Within a few years, Lo had recovered his health and had made significant strides in taijiquan. In 1974, at Professor Zheng's suggestion, Lo traveled to America, settling in San Francisco, where he has taught taijiquan for thirty-six years.

The long-running and nationally prestigious A Taste of China event, founded in 1983 by Steve Rhodes and Pat Rice and held annually for more than twenty-five years in Winchester, Virginia, honored Lo and his pushing-hands skill by naming its highest push-hands competition award (beginning in 1988) the Ben Lo Cup. The award was soon won by Lo's student, Lenzie Williams. For many years Lo has also served as a highly regarded association advisor for the Taibei Shizhong School, as well as for the Master Zheng Taijiquan Study Association, established in Taibei in 1993.

Within a year after Lo began his private taijiquan studies in Taiwan, Professor Zheng began teaching a public class, and Liu Xiheng was among the students in the first formal session. From that day in 1950, Liu and Lo developed a close relationship, not only as classmates and "brothers" in the same martial family, but also as friends. These two disciples greatly respected and faithfully served their teacher, Zheng Manqing,[8] and their warm personal friendship lasted almost six decades, up until Liu's passing in the spring of 2009.

Non-Chinese readers are encouraged to keep in mind that Mr. Lo's remarks (and those of the following three writers) were originally written and published in the context of Chinese culture and for a Chinese audience. This is an environment in which personal modesty is considered a great virtue, and its conventions of speech and writing are quite different from those of Western cultures. Therefore, meanings are sometimes difficult to translate and subtle cultural implications can easily be lost. The compiler appreciates the reader's sensitivity to this issue in the presentation of the English translation. What follows is Mr. Lo's article.

Notes

[7] For an in-depth interview with Ben Lo exploring his views and personal history, see Davis & Mann (1996). Also see the essay entitled "Ben Lo: Modest man, true taiji" in Smith (1999: 294).

[8] Professor Zheng is reported to have once commented regarding these two

outstanding and devoted students that Liu had inherited his "softness," and Lo his "fire." In other words, these two sincere disciples reflected the yin and yang elements of the master's taijiquan style respectively (Smith, 1999: 312).

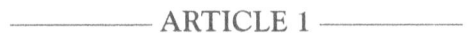
ARTICLE 1

In Memory of Brother Liu Xiheng
by Benjamin Lo • Written on April 30, 2009

On April 8 of this year (2009), I received an international call from Michael Schnapp, one of Brother Liu Xiheng's American students. He told me that Master Liu had passed away. On hearing the news, I was shocked. I had known Brother Liu Xiheng had been bedridden with sickness for some time. His initial condition was up and down, but it gradually went downhill to the point that he had to be cared for by his family because he could no longer take care of himself. However, I did not think it was that critical. I thought his condition was stable and that he would be with us for quite a while, so I was very surprised to hear that he had gone so abruptly. When I heard the bad news, I felt a surge of sorrow. I could not help but reminisce about our good times together, especially our early days in Taibei, and I reflected on our friendship as classmates for over sixty years. Like a movie, all the past seemed to flash through my mind, scene by scene.

I met Brother Liu in 1950, the year Master Zheng Manqing was invited by the mayor of Taibei, Mr. Yu Michien, to teach taiji and to promote traditional culture at Zhongshan Hall in Taibei. Brother Liu was one of the students of the first class. At the time, he was working at the executive office of the provincial food bureau, and I was just a freshman entering the National Taiwan University. There were about forty students in that taiji class. We practiced early every morning. Taiji was for him both a hobby and a means to get exercise. However, I began my study of taijiquan because of my poor health. For over a year, starting in 1948, I had been seeking medical help for my health but to no avail. The fact that I was young and yet in such poor health really worried me. At the end of 1949, when Master Zheng Manqing moved from Hong Kong to Taibei, my father took me to consult him. Master Zheng was an outstanding practitioner of traditional Chinese herbal medicine and had been the chairman of the National Chinese Medical Association in mainland China, in addition to being a professor of painting and other fine arts. His high position bespeaks his excellent medical qualifications. With the aid of his herbal prescription, my health had improved gradually, but Professor Zheng had also advised me to build up the strength of my body. In other words, he felt that I needed to practice taiji to boost my immunity. Motivated to regain my health and at the order of my physician, I plunged passionately into the practice of taijiquan without hesitation. In those early days, before the founding of his official school at Zhongshan Hall in Taibei, I practiced at Professor Zheng's private residence. Naturally, when he began teaching publicly, I also joined that first class to continue my practice and, there, I met Brother Liu Xiheng. After practicing taiji for a time, my health improved, and I have never stopped practicing since. When we had completed the whole session of the first class, some students signed up for the second class and, in addition, routinely met to practice on Sundays at Professor Zheng's house. Brother Liu was among those who never missed a practice session. Under the guidance of Master Zheng we practiced tuishou (push-hands). From then on, the Sunday gathering became our tradition no matter where Zheng lived. First, we met at Professor's old house in Xindian City (Hsintien), then at his home on Ren Ai Road, Section 3 in Taibei, and later in Yonghe City. Each and every time we met, we would spend many hours practicing till everyone was drenched with sweat, and then we would happily go our separate ways to our homes. This tradition ended only when Master Zheng moved to the USA. However, whenever Professor Zheng returned to Taiwan for a visit, the tradition would immediately resume.

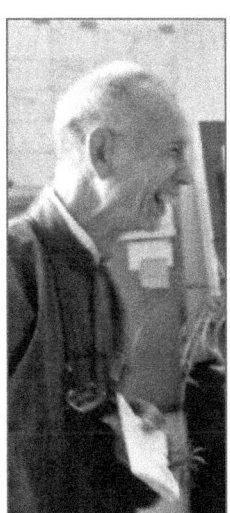 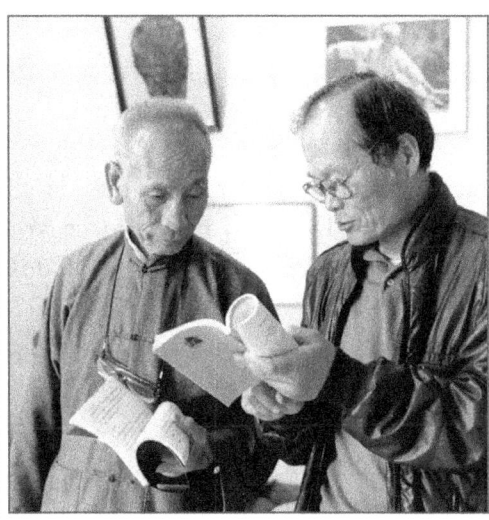 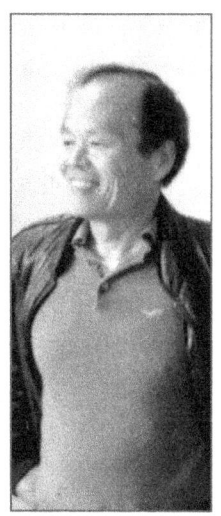

Liu and Lo examine a text under a photo of
Professor Zheng and share a lighthearted moment.
Photos courtesy of Yuan Weiming.

Time flies, and only a few of the students from that first class still survive today. As I now write these words, I feel a deep sense of the truth of the proverb that "time waits for no man." Although I am now old, I can't escape the feeling that my own efforts have amounted to nothing.

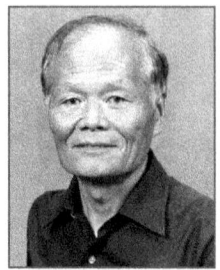

Ben Lo. Courtesy of B. Lo.

In 1953 I graduated from college. When I passed the civil service exam run by the government, I was assigned to work in the provincial government office. Fortunately, the office was located in Taibei, and did not affect my practice routine with Brother Liu. Sometimes after our Sunday practice at Professor's house, a few of us fellow students would lunch together and continue our discussion, sharing our thoughts and describing how we felt when we pushed hands with Professor Zheng. Each time, we ended our discussion with a feeling of happy camaraderie.

Brother Liu was very serious when he practiced taiji. He was extremely hard working and never missed a practice session. He was modest, gracious, and sincere to others. We developed a special relationship beyond that of classmates. He was twelve years older than I, so I respected him as an elder brother. I practiced forms and pushed hands with him a lot. However, the provincial government office where I worked soon moved to Zhong Xing New Village (Xin Cun), Nantou County, in the central part of Taiwan. I had no choice but to part from Master Zheng and all my brothers at the school and, of course, this move also interrupted my routine of practicing with Brother Liu. It was only when Brother Liu took business trips to our provincial government office that we had the occasional chance to get together. At all of those meetings, although our time together was short, we were very happy for the chance to talk with each other. One time I suggested that when we retired we should partner up and set up a school to teach taiji together because of two reasons. First, in both of our cases, our health benefited a lot from the practice of taiji, so we should share this benefit with others. Second, we were both strongly committed to passing on Master Zheng's philosophy of "spreading all goodness to others." Brother Liu totally agreed with my suggestion. What I did not know was that I would move to the USA before my retirement. My dream of teaching taiji in Taiwan did not come true, but Brother Liu's did. He taught taijiquan from the time he retired from his job with the provincial food bureau.

Regarding how I came to America, I had never thought that I would ever immigrate to the USA. My plan was to spend my remaining life in Taiwan, but who can ever know the future? In 1970 my wife was having difficulty adapting to the muggy subtropical weather of Taiwan. She was always troubled by minor health problems, so she dreamed of moving back to the USA for good. By that time, Professor Zheng had set up the US branch of his "Shr Jung" (Shizhong) Taijiquan School in New York City. My wife heard this news and was very happy, so he told me that he would love for me to come to America to help him out. I resigned from my regular job in May of 1974 and left Taiwan with my wife and our young child. The three of us moved to San Francisco, California, where I set up a school named the Universal Taijiquan Association. That started my taijiquan teaching career. The dream that I was not able to achieve in Taiwan materialized here in America. Time has passed swiftly, and thirty-five years have already flown by. Except for the first three years that I lived in America, I have traveled back to visit Taiwan almost every year. In Taiwan, I met up with my former school classmates and, of course, with Brother Liu. At every opportunity that we had to meet, he and I always exchanged stories of our personal experience teaching taiji.

In 1975, when Professor Zheng passed away, the Taibei Shizhong Taiji School founded by Master Zheng needed a successor. To ensure Professor Zheng's wishes for the continued promotion of taijiquan, Master Zheng's wife passed the leadership of the school to Brother Liu. Several years passed, and when Brother Liu found himself too old to continue to be in charge of the school, he passed the helm to Brother Xu Yizhong. The Taibei Shizhong School has thus continued operation until today. As one of the school members, I have felt ashamed that I have not been able to make a more substantial contribution. Because of this, I still feel regret.[9]

From the years I was with Brother Liu, there was one incident that I can never forget. It was the year 1950, when Master Zheng completed his book entitled *Thirteen Treatises on Taijiquan*. The manuscript was handwritten in Professor's cursive-style Chinese calligraphy. To avoid any printing errors by the publisher through possible misreading of the master's handwriting, I was asked to recopy the manuscript using standardized "printing-style" characters. When I got to the fourth treatise, "Change of personality," Master Zheng asked me what my opinion was of the article. In it Professor Zheng had written about his idea that a practitioner of the art, after going through taiji's slow, soft movements and peaceful discipline, would eventually change his or her personality. But I said frankly that I disagreed. When Master Zheng asked me why, I quoted a famous Chinese proverb, "Rivers and mountains are easy to change, but one's personality is hard to transform." (This means that, compared to changing a human being's character, it is easier to change the nation's government or the ruling dynasty—an almost impossible task.) Professor Zheng did not agree. After the book was published, Master Zheng still posed the same question to me from time to time. I stuck with my answer, so he called me "stubborn." One day, when Professor Zheng asked me about the issue again, Brother Liu came in. Master was delighted and related the question to Brother Liu for his opinion. Brother Liu said, "Master is right." Professor Zheng smilingly said, "Right, you see!" However, surprisingly, Brother Liu continued and said, "Pangjeng is also correct." At this, I gave a smile. Professor Zheng then said, "No, that can't be. You had better come up with a good explanation for saying this, or you will be in need of being disciplined by a good spanking!" Brother Liu then explained, saying, "Yes, what Master said is right because it is possible that a practitioner could somehow turn into a better, kinder person, but that does not necessarily mean a complete makeover of his personality. In this sense, Pangjeng is not wrong." I immediately expressed my agreement with this view. Professor Zheng then laughed it off and let the matter be. He never asked me about the issue ever again. When we sauntered out of Professor Zheng's house, I told Brother Liu, "Today, I have seen your ability to handle a delicate issue. I am impressed." I could have never thought of such an answer. This showed Brother Liu's penetrating insight into a matter and my relative stubbornness.[10]

Brother Liu was a lifelong believer in and follower of Buddhism. This may be why he lived to such an old age. He told me that, in his youth, he had lived like a monk but that he had later returned to a lay lifestyle.[11] However, he did practice meditation in considerable depth, and he had not stopped his practice of meditation for several decades. Now, he has passed away. I hope he is reborn in Buddha's paradise. As Chan (Zen) Master Pu Chao, a monk of the Yuan dynasty, once said, "Being released from the mundane world, he has returned to nature; on that day such a one has passed on ahead of us to his next life alone."[12]

(End of Benjamin Lo's article)

Notes

[9] The compiler of this article would like to note that, while Mr. Lo's expression of regret is most certainly sincere, his comment is an example of the virtue of Chinese modesty and humility. Mr. Lo has traveled to Taiwan many times since 1974 and has made important contributions to Professor's school and legacy there, as well as in America. Where a Western writer might focus on his own accomplishments, Mr. Lo chooses not to do so. Instead, he focuses on the lack.

[10] This is yet another case of Mr. Lo exemplifying the virtue of humility. Mr. Lo's

purpose here is to praise Mr. Liu and to highlight his wisdom and intelligence, not to praise himself. Mr. Liu was able to skillfully resolve the disagreement between master and disciple by taking the middle path between two extreme positions, stubbornly held, thus upholding both Confucian and Buddhist values and preserving face for both parties.

11 As a youth, Liu lived for a time in Nanshan Temple in Xiamen (Amoy) with his older cousin, who was a Buddhist monk. Liu was sometimes called upon to read sutras and had frequent interactions and friendships with monks, including the famous Hong Yi (Li Shutong) of Nanputou Temple. After his schooling, he married, raised a family, and pursued a career as a civil servant. However, later in life Liu committed himself deeply to the practice of Buddhist meditation as a lay practitioner.

12 Pu Chao was a famous Chan master (Chin., *channa*; Sanskrit, *dhyana*; Jap. Zen, after *zazen*, or sitting meditation; i.e., Pu Chao was a master of Buddhist meditation) and monk of the Yuan dynasty (1279–1368 CE). The quotation attributed to him and applied here to Mr. Liu is meant to refer to one who has attained a very high level of insight into "Buddha mind," "original nature," or "fundamental reality." The gist of the quote is that such a person is without peer.

Introduction to Xu Yizhong's Memorial Article

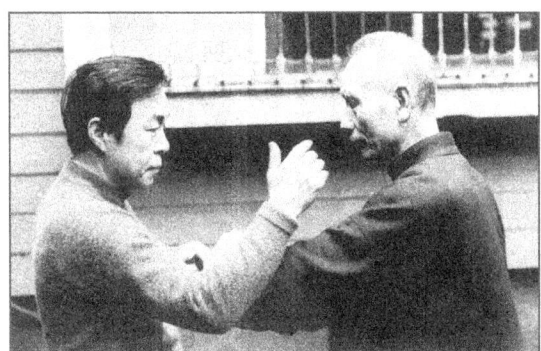

Xu Yizhong (left) and Liu Xiheng (right).
Photograph by Hsiao Peihsien from
Evergreen Magazine, Issue #14, 1984.

Xu Yizhong is a well-known disciple of Zheng Manqing. He has done much to promote his master's style of taijiquan, especially in Taiwan but also in China. Xu began his studies with Zheng at the same time Liu did, as a member of Zheng's first public class on the island. Xu succeeded his "martial arts brother," Liu, as head of

Zheng's Shizhong School (known in Taiwan as the Shizhong Study Society) in Taibei at the time of Liu's retirement from that position in 1986 and continues to head the school today. In 1993 Xu was elected first committee chairman of a new organization, the Master Zheng Taijiquan Study Association. Chairman Xu served the first two consecutive terms of this new post, up until 1999. After brief terms served by Ke Qihua and Ju Hongbin, Xu returned to the post and continued to serve until his retirement in 2008, when he was succeeded by Fu Kunhe.

In addition to holding these important positions and training several generations of students in Zheng's lineage in Taiwan, in 2005 Xu traveled to Nankai University in Tianjin, China, where he had been invited to reintroduce Professor Zheng's thirty-seven-posture Yang-style short form to students on the mainland. More than seven decades prior, Professor Zheng had taught taijiquan at the Central Military Academy (formerly known as Huangpu) in 1933 and at the provincial government's Hunan Martial Arts Academy in 1938 (Davis, 1996: 41). It was at the latter, while given only two months' time to train hundreds of officers, that Zheng had first experimented with shortening the traditional long Yang form that he had inherited from his teacher, Yang Chengfu (Cheng, 1965/1999: 9; Mason, 2008: 25–26, 37; Wile, 2007: 80, 103–104). Finally, Xu played a major role in the establishment and continued operation of the Zheng Manqing Memorial Hall, located at Zheng's former Taiwan residence in Yonghe City, just south of Taibei City (Mason, 2008: 30). What follows is Mr. Xu's article.

———————— ARTICLE 2 ————————

A Salute to Brother Liu Xiheng
by Xu Yizhong • Written in May of 2009

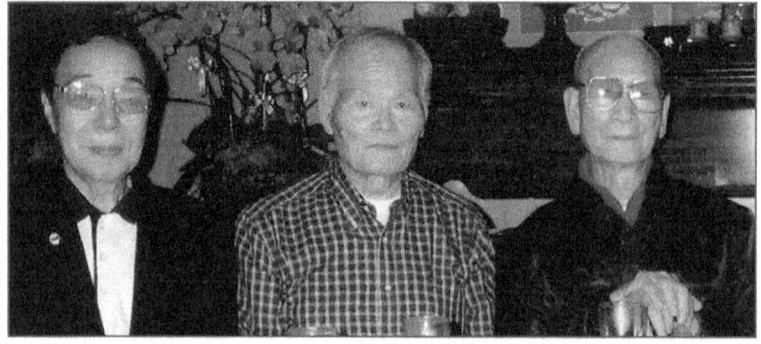

Xu, Lo, and Liu at a banquet in Taibei (December 2004).
Photo courtesy of Danny Emerick.

My eldest school brother, Liu Xiheng, was kind hearted and honest. A lifelong believer and practitioner of Buddhism, he also practiced taijiquan diligently and was very healthy. Unfortunately, he passed away in April of 2009. He died in Taiwan University Hospital in Taibei and, at the time of his passing, was ninety-five years of age. He is survived by many children and grandchildren. This is what we call the "fulfillment of life and fortune."

I met Brother Liu in the winter of 1949, when we both attended the first taiji class founded by Master Zheng Manqing after his arrival in Taiwan. The class was held in Zhongshan Hall in the city of Taibei. Although it has been sixty years, I can still recall that our class consisted of about fifty students. Brother Liu often mingled among us and assisted the master with administrative affairs. Due to his warm and modest personality and his enthusiastic attitude toward service, he was well respected by his classmates. Studying together day in and day out, we found each other to have a lot in common. We were very close; we kept no secrets from one another, nor did we ever run out of topics of conversation. His knowledge and experience were way ahead of me, so I benefited a lot from our relationship. Now that he is gone, we can only fall back on our memories of those old times. Here, I would like to share two incidents that may not be known by many people. This will serve as my memorial to my old friend.

(1) There was a book written by Master Zheng Manqing entitled *An Interpretation of the Analects of Confucius*. Brother Liu was assigned to rewrite the text in standard calligraphy in order to prepare it for printing. After the job was completed, Brother Liu saved the original handwritten manuscript and stored it in a box for decades. When Master Zheng passed away, knowing that this could be of value and that it was a precious legacy of the master, he asked how it should be disposed of. He intended to return it to Master's wife, but I suggested that, since she was living in the USA, we should keep it as our heirloom. However, Brother Liu insisted that we should return it to Master Zheng's wife. I am a witness that he did exactly that when she visited Taiwan the next year.

(2) Brother Liu was appointed to work in the provincial food bureau for decades when he moved from mainland China to Taiwan. His position was at the top level of public servants. On his annual job evaluations he was rated excellent every year. In 1976 the chief minister of the food bureau had to be reappointed to a new position as the general secretariat of the bureau. According to agency policy, Brother Liu should have been able to retain his position; however, as the positions of general secretariat and vice minister were being reappointed, the personnel office had a dilemma as to how to deal with Liu's positioning. Brother Liu heard about the situation and immediately announced his early retirement, thereby resolving the predicament of the newly appointed

minister and the personnel office. His courage and willingness to sacrifice himself for the good of others should be a model for all public servants nowadays.

(End of Xu Yizhong's article)

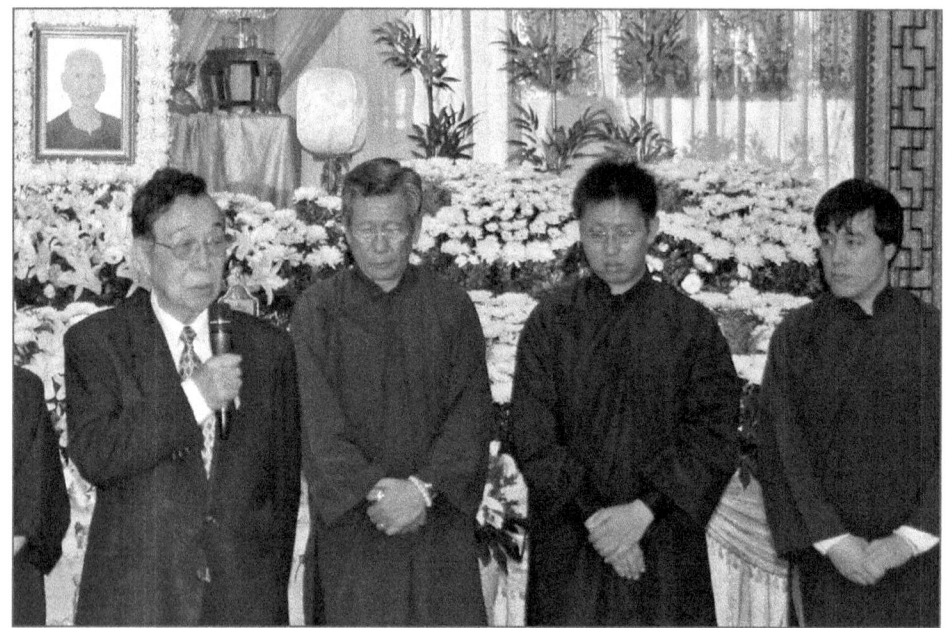

Xu (on left) with mourners at Liu's funeral.
Photo courtesy of Yuan Weiming.

Introduction to Yuan Weiming's Memorial Article

The author of the following article, Yuan Weiming, is a disciple of Liu Xiheng, having studied with the master since receiving a formal introduction in 1982. Previously, while pursuing graduate studies in the United States at Washington University, Yuan had studied taijiquan with other senior students of Professor Zheng Manqing, and he cofounded the St. Louis T'ai Chi Ch'uan Association in 1978. Four years later he returned to Taiwan, became a disciple of Liu, and intensified his training. Yuan subsequently accompanied his master on his overseas trips in the late eighties, serving as his translator and teaching assistant. He has worked for many years as an instructor and coach for the Taibei Shizhong Taijiquan School (a.k.a., the Shizhong Study Society), is a professional photographer, and is a professor of architecture and design at Tunghai University in Taichung, Taiwan. Yuan regularly travels to the US to conduct taijiquan training workshops in the tradition of Professor Zheng and Master Liu. What follows is Yuan Weiming's article.

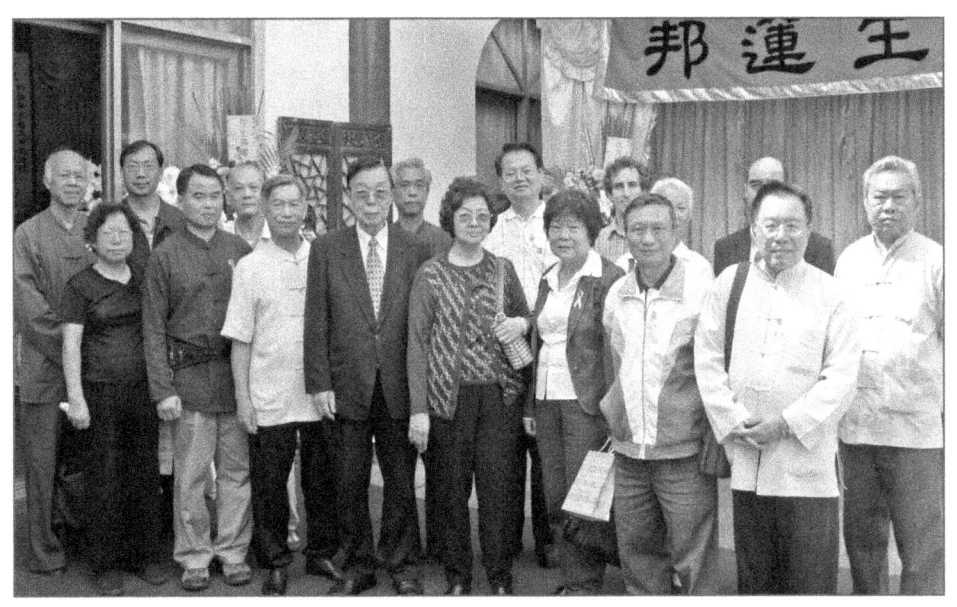

Mourners at Liu's funeral. Standing at far left:
Professor Yuan Weiming; seventh from the left
in coat and tie: President Xu Yizhong.

———————— ARTICLE 3 ————————

In Memory of Liu Laoshi
by Yuan Weiming • Written on October 8, 2009

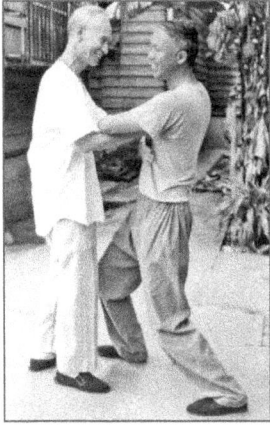

Liu and Yuan push hands.
Photo courtesy of Yuan Weiming.

My respected teacher, Mr. Liu Xiheng (addressed as Laoshi by his students), left us in the spring of 2009 on April 8. He had expected to live only as long as his teacher, Professor Zheng Manqing, but he ended up living twenty years longer. Laoshi's passing brought deep sorrow and a sense of loss to his wife, his family, his taijiquan friends and colleagues, and his students. The regret he felt when he lost his own beloved teacher has now pierced our hearts.

At this time, I think the most meaningful thing I can do to honor the memory of Laoshi is to help people within the taiji community know Mr. Liu better by revealing some of the personal character of this great teacher. It is with this idea in mind that I record these words. In a certain sense, this article has been written by Laoshi himself for, besides some impressions and memories from my personal experience, most of the words used here are his. I have merely reorganized the words of Laoshi's own instructional narrative.

In 1982 I returned to Taiwan after a time of study in the US. Through the recommendation of Mr. Benjamin Pangjeng Lo, I was able to study taijiquan with Mr. Liu. At that time, the classes were held at his personal residence, and this period is also the most memorable time of my studies. The house actually belonged to the Bureau of Provisions, but it was assigned to Laoshi when he worked there as the head secretary of the bureau. It was a walled, Japanese-style bungalow with a red door, located in a quiet alley of Taibei. The little courtyard of the house only allowed space for about ten people to practice taijiquan. In order to be nearby, I also moved into an apartment on the same alley.

I took part in the morning class. The usual three-hour session started with the students and Laoshi performing the taiji form together; then we practiced some basic movements developed by Laoshi and, finally, Laoshi would take turns doing push-hands (tuishou) with each student in the class. In between, Laoshi would talk about taiji theory or tell us anecdotes related to taijiquan.

Early in the morning, before the class started, Laoshi always took time to prepare a pot of tea for his students, but I hardly ever saw Laoshi sit down and drink tea; he was the only one in the class who never took a break. There were some fruit trees and flowers planted in the courtyard garden. During the class, Laoshi would sometimes pause to walk aside and smell the jasmine flowers, and he would also invite us to pluck the loquats and bananas from the nearby trees. While practicing, we often saw Laoshi's youngest daughter rushing past on her way to work and his mischievous grandson playing around in the courtyard. From time to time, the class was interrupted by unexpected visitors, most of whom were people from the taijiquan circle. During this morning routine, a joyful mood filled the whole place. Laoshi was always smiling when he pushed hands with his students, as if he were playing a game with great amusement. This childlike character, in my opinion, reflects Laoshi's true nature. It was within this environment that we gradually became better acquainted with the art of taijiquan.

Unfortunately, I was only able to study in this idyllic setting for six years. The house was finally torn down and an apartment building was erected on the site. What I missed most was the garage wall where we practiced push-hands. The wall had become soaked with the sweat of many toiling students, and the surface was covered with the words of instruction that Laoshi had written with a fragment of brick while instructing us during class. After he moved from the house, our class subsequently met in several different locations, including a rooftop site and a local park. Finally, we settled in on the grounds of a nearby university campus. Although the class atmosphere never changed, the environment of these later locations was not as moving. Those of us who studied in that tiny courtyard will always remember the inspirational force of this mixture of family life and teaching.

When considering whether to accept a student, the only condition Mr. Liu required was that he (or she) have a respectful attitude. Therefore, he rejected people who just wanted to have a taste of what the class was like and who were not committed to the study of the art. Similarly, he rejected those who came only to test his ability. Sincerity was all that was required; talent was insignificant. The amount of the tuition also depended on a student's personal financial situation. The attitude of sincerity was shown mutually; Mr. Liu also paid the same respect to his students. Laoshi had a theory about this: "Only through sincere teaching and learning can the highest level of taijiquan skill be developed." More often than not, we felt Laoshi offered more sincerity and diligence to his students than we gave him. Once a person had become his student, whether a formal disciple or not, Laoshi would teach without differentiation, and he always taught personally; he never relied on his senior students, even to instruct beginners. The teaching was offered solely in the group-class environment. Laoshi hardly ever gave any private lessons. No matter how much tuition was offered to him, he remained unmoved. Due to his personal example, Laoshi's students were all respectful to one another.

Throughout my years of studying with Mr. Liu, one thing that impressed me greatly was the continuous stream of foreign students visiting from all over the world. Some students stayed weeks, some stayed months, some tried to find jobs and settle down, and some even got married and started families. Perhaps due to the cultural difference, foreign students were particularly fascinated by this special relationship between teacher and students; they respected Laoshi as a mentor and, sometimes, as a father figure. One student even became his foster son. And one of his earliest disciples from America continued to write to Laoshi for about twenty-five years—even though Laoshi did not write him back. Laoshi's only foreign female disciple, Lin Farley, although lacking contact information and not being proficient in the Chinese language, traveled to mainland China, found Laoshi's hometown, and located his relatives. Her efforts to help him reestablish contact with his family pleased Laoshi very much. Later, after Lin left Taiwan and lost contact with her teacher, Laoshi never ceased looking for her.

Mr. Liu's emphasis on loyalty and sincerity was apparently derived from his own loyalty to his teacher, Professor Zheng Manqing. He was among the earliest group of disciples, and, of all Professor Zheng's followers, Mr. Liu spent more time in class with the Professor than any other student. From the time that he first took Professor's class in 1949, he never stopped learning from him. For example, Professor Zheng taught taiji sword only three times in Taiwan, and Mr. Liu was the only student who was present for all three courses of instruction. Because of Laoshi's honesty, earnestness, and integrity, Professor trusted him very much. He started as a student but gradually became a trusted assistant, helping to handle accounting and proofreading duties. Eventually, he became the senior-most disciple and was asked to lead form practice as a model for the other students from a position at the front of the class.

Laoshi often quoted a sentence from the classical writings of the Daoist philosopher Zhuangzi to express his idea about the proper relationship between a teacher and a student: "When the teacher walks, I follow him walking; when the teacher walks faster, I also walk faster, trying to catch up with him." The loyalty and trust that Laoshi felt toward Professor Zheng were genuine, without the slightest doubt. He said: "Faith is the same as religious belief; the faith that is generated from sincerity can produce wonderful things."

Shortly before his death in 1975, Professor Zheng came back to Taiwan from New York, and the whole class gathered at a banquet in his honor. One student asked Professor: "If you, our master, were not around, who should lead us? Professor pointed to Mr. Liu and said, "Just him." Madame Zheng and the students regarded this event as Professor's appointment of his successor: the "gatekeeper" (*zhang men ren*) of the school, but Laoshi never thought of the matter in this way. His attitude and behavior were as usual, without showing any change or influence from this incident. This reflects his modest demeanor and demonstrates the quality of "no-self" sought by devotees of the Buddhist dharma. After Professor's passing and Mr. Liu's official appointment as head of the Shizhong Society, a position he held from 1975 until 1986, Laoshi continued to exhibit this quality of character.

Mr. Liu always kept a low profile in the public arena. He never brought students with him to perform at public demonstrations, or desired to publish any magazine articles about taijiquan [see footnote #5], and he certainly did not care about things that happened in taijiquan circles. Even in regard to his teaching of taijiquan, he never endeavored to promote it widely; therefore, he had no intention of recruiting a large group of followers and cared nothing about fame. Because of his humble attitude, he remained a somewhat obscure figure in the world of taiji. He only concentrated on teaching a small group of dedicated students. After he resigned from his position as the president of the Shizhong Society, except for an occasional lecture appearance at Shizhong and the teaching of his small class of disciples and students, he had hardly any contact with the outside world. The only thing he concerned himself with was the art of taijiquan itself, and he would accept any theory or idea as long as it was beneficial to the practice of taijiquan.

For Laoshi, taijiquan was a way of self-cultivation and of obtaining wisdom and guidance for life; the martial arts applications were only a minor aspect of the art. For that reason, he did not like to be called "Master" because that conflicted with his beliefs. The best way to exemplify this idea is by describing his attitude toward push-hands. He regarded the push-hands practice as being about learning to be a better human being—in other words, learning to establish good interactions with others. When we practiced push-hands, he instructed us to just calm the mind and to concentrate on "listening to" the movements of the opponent (ting jin). Even if a student had developed good listening and neutralization skills and was able to push his partner, he was to resist the temptation to push. Instead, he was to continue to "follow" until his partner had lost all opportunity to advance. In this way, we would not only learn the skill of pushing hands, but we would also cultivate ourselves and develop the qualities of endurance, composedness, and stabilization of the energy (qi) and the mind (yi). Our focus was to be on cultivating ourselves rather than on overcoming an opponent.

He often repeated the phrase, "Let yourself be untouchable, and don't try to be unmovable." Yielding is always the highest principle. Even when the opponent has committed a fault by using force, one should only pay attention to one's own movements and not try to blame the other person. When he pushed hands with students, Laoshi also followed his own principle. Although he was capable of neutralizing and pushing the student out in every move, he always neutralized several times before he pushed the student away, and even when he did so, it was with a very light touch. The push was just enough to cause the student to lose his balance. He pushed "hard" only when the student was using excessive force or when a student was about to leave the class and travel far away.[13] It seemed that he wanted the student to keep the memory of this feeling of being pushed with correct, clear technique. Only at that moment did we get to witness the tremendous power Laoshi possessed. Mr. Ben Lo once advised him that, at his advanced age, he should not practice push-hands anymore, but Laoshi insisted on continuing to practice with his students. However, as he got older, he sought only to relax and neutralize, not to push.

With this kind of mentality and attitude, I think Mr. Liu had developed a very pure and refined taijiquan art, and only someone who has studied taijiquan for a long time can understand and appreciate the value of this kind of achievement in the art. Several senior students of Professor Zheng in Taiwan (e.g., Xu Yizhong, Ke Qihua, Su Shaoqing, and Chen Youyi) as well as from the US (e.g., Ed Young, Maggie Newman, Robert W. Smith, Carol Yamasaki, and Wolfe Lowenthal) came to Laoshi asking for instruction. Everyone who had pushed hands with Laoshi gave a very high evaluation of his skills. One person said he was like an "agile snake." The late David Chen said trying to push Laoshi felt like pushing with an empty jacket on a hanger. Perhaps the most valuable comments came from several students of Professor from abroad, who claimed that the feeling of pushing with Mr. Liu was the closest to the experience of pushing with Professor Zheng. Laoshi was contented with his regular routine and simple life. Although he was invited many times to teach abroad, he only agreed twice, traveling to Holland and the US in 1987 and 1988, and a good portion of his reason for going on these occasions was to enjoy the experience of traveling abroad with his wife. After Mrs. Liu was unable to travel far, he rejected all subsequent invitations to do foreign teaching.

Despite his high achievement in taijiquan, Laoshi insisted that he would not write any books or make any films. When his students asked him to leave us some visual images, he just said: "I am still in progress; do you want me to stop progressing?" Sometimes he would add: "Taijiquan is about the internal and not the external; you should not rely too much on images of the external structure." One time when he was talking about this matter, he said: "I follow Confucius: 'Talk, but do not write.'" The hidden meaning of this statement is that writing is for a luminary, like Professor Zheng, to do. Laoshi considered himself to be just a follower; to propagate the master's teachings was enough for him. Sometimes he would pause in the middle of making a comment about taijiquan. When we asked him why, he would say: "Buddha said, 'It cannot be put into words.'" In profound matters, the more you talk about it, the more confusion will be generated. To extend that idea, in his later days, Laoshi often said that his taijiquan is a "hard but casual" way of practice. Not too many people can comprehend the true meaning of that statement.[14] It is unfortunate that today we only have a few photographs and recordings of lectures to recall Mr. Liu's presence. Most of his teachings existed only immaterially in the form of his oral presentations, and precious images of Laoshi are stored only in the memories of his students.

For Mr. Liu, two essential aspects of taijiquan were to apply the principles of the art to daily life and to join them with the tenets of Buddhism. Many years ago, when Professor Zheng was still in the US, in one of their exchanges of correspondence, Laoshi complained about his heavy workload. Professor replied and upbraided him with these words: "Where is your practice of sinking the qi down to the dantian?" Laoshi suddenly realized that taijiquan had to be practiced in daily life and, from then on, he followed his teacher's admonition and worked hard on that concept. Besides using the principles of push-hands to practice how to deal with other people and to cultivate the virtue of modesty, Laoshi also sometimes quoted a phrase from the taijiquan *Classics* to respond to the questions students asked concerning the various situations that happen in life. For example, when pursuing a relationship with a girlfriend, one should, "Stick, connect, adhere, and follow; do not detach, do not use force." Again, the way to a happy marriage is to, "Give up your self-will, and follow the other person." These words of advice usually made people smile.

Laoshi had first encountered and practiced Buddhism at a very early age, and he finally committed himself to it at the age of forty-nine. After his retirement, studying Buddhism and taijiquan became his two major tasks. Yet, he considered these two paths to be leading to the same end: peace of mind. He thought that after practicing either "way" and reaching a certain level, one could gain insight into one's own true nature. For this reason, he often used Buddhist doctrines to interpret taijiquan and used taijiquan principles to comprehend Buddhism. He used the Buddhist idea "look through and let go" to describe relaxing (song), and the notion "follow fate but remain unchanged" to explain the concept of central equilibrium (*zhong ding*). Moreover, he compared the teaching of taijiquan with "the contribution of the dharma." The words and proverbs of Buddhism were also frequently used to interpret the profound aspects of taijiquan.[15]

Laoshi was not a man of worldly desires; his character was illuminated from inside, and the people who were touched by him were not limited to those in the field of taijiquan. More than twenty years ago, when he accepted his first group of disciples, he wrote a manuscript on the importance of respecting one's teacher and sticking to the Dao. One of the disciples, who is an American and who also studied Buddhism in Taiwan, showed this manuscript to his Buddhist teacher, Master Shengyan (Zhang Baokang, 1930–2009), a very famous Buddhist monk in Taiwan. After looking at the essay, the master said: "Oh, there still is such a person in Taiwan! I want to meet him." He then arranged a dinner appointment with Mr. Liu, but Laoshi was detained by an unforeseen matter, and so they never had the opportunity to meet. After many years had gone by, both Master Shengyan and Laoshi passed away within a two-month interval, and they were both buried in Dharma Drum Mountain. Their fates were connected and so, in this way, they finally "met" each other.

One morning three years ago, my elder classmate, Mr. Jiang, and I went to Laoshi's apartment, which was the last place where classes were held. There Laoshi shared his final state of mind with us. He said that, a few days before, he had not been able to sleep; his mind had been disturbed by the thought that his life was approaching its end. Suddenly, he remembered the words that the famous Buddhist monk, Master Hong Yi [1880–1942], had written down before he died: "Sorrow and joy are mixed together." On thinking of that, he was enlightened and his mind became clear. We say "sorrow" because life basically is full of suffering and pain, but there is also "joy" as one contemplates his soon approaching departure for the Buddhist paradise. Laoshi has now finally fulfilled his wish. Even though we may not be willing to accept his departure, we should give him our blessing.

(End of Yuan Weiming's article)

Notes

[13] Sometimes it felt to the student that Laoshi "pushed powerfully," but it was only because the student himself was using excessive force (i.e., Laoshi then allowed the student's own force to return to him).

[14] The statement: "*Ma ma, hu hu*" usually means "doesn't care much; perfunctory." What Mr. Liu meant more profoundly is, "Your mind should be relaxed; don't care too much about loss and gain; don't try to push others; don't worry about your gongfu achievement . . . ." Laoshi also told the compiler of this article, "If you try to pin it down too definitely, to grasp it tightly with your mind, you will only push it further away. You must relax and use your intuition to grasp the essence with your heart." Also, Danny Emerick remembers Laoshi saying laughingly that taiji was "simple but not easy."

[15] Though a number of Master Liu's students had an interest in Buddhism, Laoshi seemed to respect our individual paths and faith traditions and did not push us to follow him in that direction.

Introduction to Xu Zhengmei's Memorial Article

The fourth of the memorial articles was written by Xu Zhengmei, a disciple of Liu Xiheng and a retired teacher of mathematics formerly employed by Jianguo High School, Taibei, Taiwan. Xu's primary purpose is to provide some brief biographical material on Liu. He also includes a poem he composed, providing a fitting touch to this memorial project.

ARTICLE 4

A Brief Biography of Mr. Liu Xiheng
by Xu Zhengmei • Written in 2009

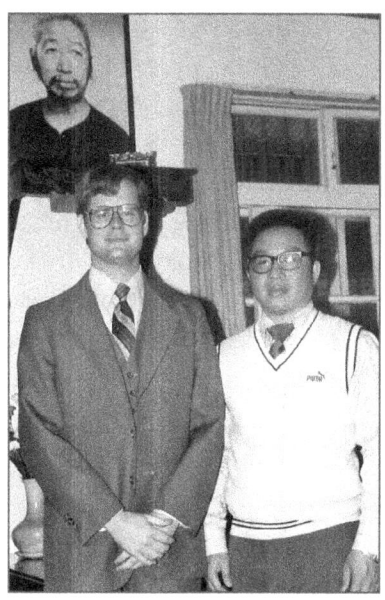

Danny Emerick and Xu Zhengmei at Professor
Zheng's home (1984). Photo courtesy of D. Emerick.

Mr. Liu Xiheng was born on December 10, 1915, in Raoping County, Guandong Province. He was the youngest child of his family and, since there were four sisters and five brothers before him, he was the "number ten" child. His father was a fisherman and, although his family was poor, they were happy and contented.

In his teens Liu attended elementary school in Xiamen (Amoy) City with his older cousin, who was a Buddhist monk. Liu lodged and dined in the Nanshan Temple with his cousin. Leading a disciplined life of temple routine, he felt happy. His intellectual giftedness was manifested by his high achievement at school in spite of adversity. However, that was a time of warlords and social upheaval, as well as the Japanese invasion, so his schooling was interrupted many times. His education proceeded sporadically during his junior high, high school, and college years; however, he never gave up pursuing higher studies, even though he had to continue with self-study during periods when he was not able to attend formal classes. In this way he managed to pass his entrance exams at each and every step, from middle school to college. He was a person of diligence and superb intelligence.

After only a year and a half of high school, he was forced to discontinue his formal studies due to poor health. While recuperating in Nanshan Temple, he bought a book entitled *Taiji: A Scientific Approach*, by Wu Tunan. Through self-study he practiced taijiquan according to the instructions contained in this book. Within a year his health improved. Then he passed the qualifying exam for Amoy University and was enrolled into its Department of Economics. When he had difficulty covering his costs for college, his teacher came to his aid and provided financial assistance. During his college days, he found time to continue his practice of taijiquan in a quiet corner of the campus. One day, the head of the Physical Education Department discovered his ability in taiji and hired him as an assistant to teach the students taijiquan. This was during the Sino-Japanese War, and a majority of the students were suffering from malnutrition and poor health due to inadequate food supplies. Liu was paid for the job, which was a cause of great excitement for him. This small stipend helped him to pay his way through four years of college. During his winter and summer breaks, he also taught Mandarin to the young monks in Nanputouo Temple. There he had the opportunity to befriend Hong Yi Fashi ("Master of the Law," Monk Hong Yi). In 1942 Liu graduated, receiving his degree from Amoy University.

At the end of the war, Taiwan was liberated from Japan. The whole island needed to be rebuilt, and that great task required qualified people from all walks of life. Mr. Liu traveled to Taiwan with his wife and children and was immediately hired by the provincial food bureau. Due to his training in economic theory and his literary proficiency, he was soon appointed the secretariat and was also given a post as a special committee member for the bureau. He worked closely with the minister of the food bureau, serving as his planner. Because of his well-disciplined and no-nonsense attitude and because he could be depended upon to execute his affairs promptly and fairly, he was greatly loved by his coworkers. In 1976 he retired from the bureau.

In the winter of 1949 Professor Zheng Manqing, fourth-generation successor of the Yang-style of taijiquan, was invited by Taibei Mayor Yu Michien to start a teaching program of taijiquan in Zhongshan Hall. The school was officially named the Shizhong Taijiquan School, and Master Zheng became the chairman. At that time Mr. Liu Xiheng enrolled himself as a student in the first class, and he continued to practice Master Zheng's method of taijiquan for the rest of his life, giving him almost six decades of experience in the style. He was well acquainted with all the students of the first class, which included Liang Tongcai, Yin Qitang, Ye Xiuting, Tao Bingxiang, Ju Hongbin, Benjamin Lo, and Xu Yizhong. Benjamin Lo and Xu Yizhong were two of his best friends. After studying with Professor Zheng Manqing, Liu concluded: "Master Zheng is the real thing; in my past self-study and self-practice at Amoy University, I was using too much force, so I had been wasting the time of others and my own time as well."

Mr. Liu practiced taijiquan diligently during his spare time, and he applied the philosophy of taiji to his life as well. Because of his high intelligence and virtue, Master Zheng valued him highly, and he was appointed as master's first disciple after the founding of the Shizhong Taijiquan School. In the 1960s, while living in the USA, Master Zheng left Mr. Liu in charge of the Taibei school. The master also kept up correspondence with him in regard to the philosophy, theory, and technique of taiji. Master Zheng had high hopes for Mr. Liu.

On March 26, 1975, while visiting Taiwan, Master Zheng Manqing passed away. One year later, Mr. Liu was appointed chairman of the Taibei Shizhong Taijiquan School and was made officially responsible for carrying on the legacy of Master Zheng's Dao. Every Sunday Mr. Liu gathered all the Shizhong School brothers, and they practiced together on the campus of the Taiwan University School of Law, which was located at Xuzhou (Hsu Chou) Road. In March of 1983 he initiated the first session of Master Zheng's Taijiquan Study Class. Each session lasted six months; and thus, the training of a new class of talented students was begun. Mr. Liu was the head coach for each session of form training, as well as the leader of the push-hands group, and Mr. Xu Yizhong served as the general manager. All the coaches were selected from among the top-notch school graduates, and new students were recommended to the program by the previous graduates. This opened the door for the systematic training of a new generation of skilled Shizhong graduates and instructors.

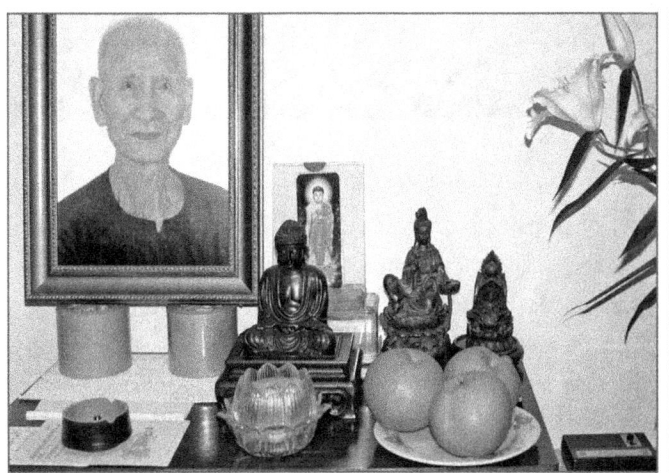
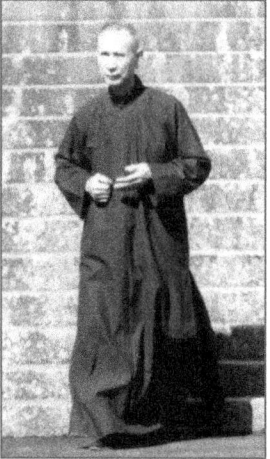

Mr. Liu's funeral portrait with Buddhist
imagery and in formal attire at a temple site.

In 1988, at the age of seventy-seven, Mr. Liu retired and passed the school leadership to Xu Yizhong. From that time, Liu led a peaceful life, concentrating on the practice and teaching of taijiquan to a small group of dedicated students and leading a lifestyle of vegetarianism and Buddhist meditation.

In 1987 and 1988 he travelled to Europe and the USA, teaching taijiquan. Mr. Liu's taiji technique was excellent. In particular, his push-hands skills of neutralization and discharge were profound and varied. Hence, he attracted the interest of a number of foreign students. However, Liu picked his students with scrupulous care. His first requirement was that a student be of virtuous character. He taught his students not only taijiquan but also the taiji philosophy of life. He always said, "The true application of taiji is to cultivate a calm spirit, a peaceful heart, and a clear and logical mind. These qualities contribute to a peaceful society."

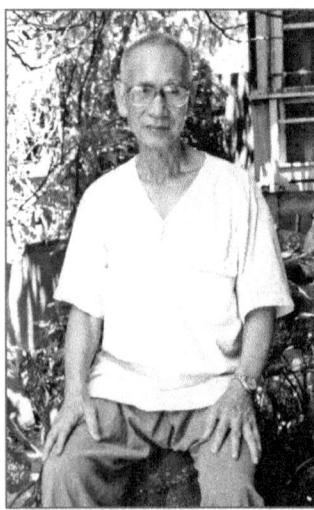 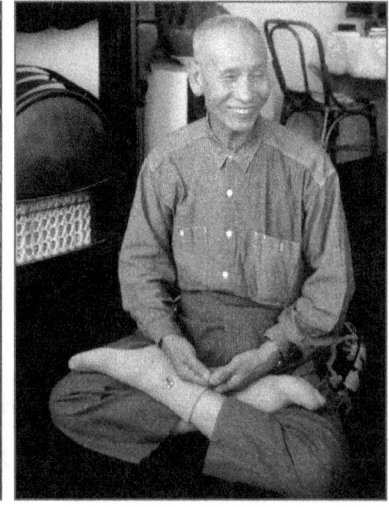 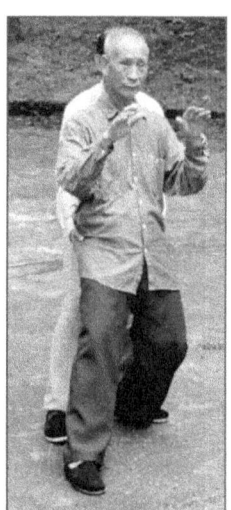

Left: Liu in a restful moment.
Center, he prepares for sitting meditation.
Right: Liu allows a student to feel
the correct position of the hips
in rear-loaded posture.
Photos courtesy of Yuan Weiming.

Now that Mr. Liu has passed away, his students and associates continue to respect him deeply and to miss him very much. I would like to remember him with the following poem, summing up Mr. Liu's way of life and his achievement in old age.

A great taiji master of his time;
For whom had he been working so diligently?
He passed the torch of Shizhong,
And he planted a garden full of fragrance.
Trees he nurtured have grown to become pillars.
He committed his whole life to
the principles of honesty, frugality, and simplicity.
A life that valued dedication and was oblivious to vainglory
Can also be considered glorious.

(End of Xu Zhengmei's article)

Introduction to Danny Emerick's Memorial Article

The fifth article is an original piece composed in English specifically for this memorial project by an American disciple of Liu Xiheng. Mr. Emerick's knowledge and experience in the Asian martial arts is extensive. He began his study of Zheng's thirty-seven-posture Yang taijiquan short form in the 1970s in the US and moved to Taibei, Taiwan, in 1981 to continue his training under Liu's tutelage. In 1982 Emerick was among the first group of Western students to be accepted as indoor disciples through a traditional *bai shi* ceremony. Today Mr. Emerick is reference librarian at the State Library of Florida in Tallahassee. His memoir brings a Western perspective to the experience of studying with Liu Xiheng. What follows is Danny Emerick's article.

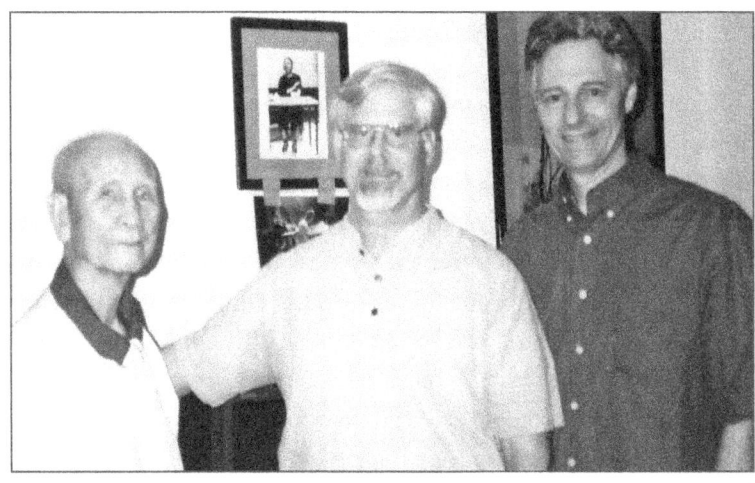

Liu Xiheng with Danny Emerick (center)
and Russ Mason (right).

——————— ARTICLE 5 ———————

A Garden of Memories
by Danny Emerick • Written on April 11, 2010

I met Mr. Liu in August 1981, but only after an exhausting twenty-four hours of travel on a plane (only my second time on an airplane), a confiscation of contraband items by the ROC customs agent (the "friend" who was to meet me at the airport neglected to tell me that the professional grade walkie-talkies that he asked me to bring from the USA were illegal to "import" under Taiwan's then somewhat strict martial law!), and surviving a car crash (coincidentally driven by that same "friend") ten minutes after leaving the Chiang Kai-shek International Airport. The crash completely totaled the car, and could have resulted in an all-too-brief stay for me on Ilha Formosa (not to mention my stay on planet earth), but miraculously left us unscathed!

So, after a few days of recovering from jetlag and jangled nerves (and from a mild case of whiplash) at the International House on Xingyi Road, I figured I was ready to meet Mr. Liu. I asked a Chinese friend (not the driver!) to call the number I had for Mr. Liu to inquire about class times and was told that there was a class the next morning at 7:30.

Mind you, I didn't know anything about Mr. Liu, only that he was recommended to me by Mr. Ben Lo (Professor Zheng Manqing's senior student) when I asked him about taiji teachers in Taibei, and that Mr. Lo would write a letter of introduction and send it to Mr. Liu so he would be expecting me. Mr. Lo also added that if he did not write this letter of introduction, Mr. Liu would probably not be inclined to teach me.

So the next day at 7:00 a.m., on a warm summer morning typical for that part of the world, I ventured out onto the streets of Taibei, armed with the address (written in Chinese, of course) of Mr. Liu Xiheng.

After consulting a map of the city and walking a few blocks, I realized that I had no idea how to decipher the address that had been given to me and desperately needed help to locate the class. This realization—intensified by the cacophony of street traffic and the bombardment of the senses by the new sights, sounds, smells and general chaos that a newcomer finds in Taibei—stopped me cold. I did what any other foreigner would do in the same situation: I panicked and accosted the next passerby who looked of college age. My Taiwanese friends back in the US told me all college students in Taiwan could speak English. Well, not quite all, I found out.

The unfortunate victim I chose did indeed look like a typical college-age student, but when I thrust the address under his nose and asked, in my best English, for his help in finding the address, instead of hearing, "Sure, no problem," I only got gestures and grins from him. The gestures seemed to be for me to follow him, however, and the grins, I suppose, were meant to be reassuring to me. They weren't. He turned down a little lane off the main road with the address in his hand and with me right behind him!

After walking down the lane for about fifteen or twenty minutes, I was growing more suspicious by the minute as to exactly what my newfound companion was really up to. He stopped in front of a red door imbedded into a seven-foot wall and pointed to the address in his hand and then to the door. Handing the paper back to me, he then turned back to continue the journey I had so rudely interrupted. But as he left he smiled a real smile, as I tried to stammer out an inadequate "thank you" that did not even begin to repay his genuine kindness to a hopelessly lost foreigner.

Whoever he was, I can only pray that he is well for if it hadn't been for this good Samaritan, I would probably still be wandering around the streets of Taibei!

Now, therefore, completely trusting the integrity of my new "friend" to have led me to the correct address, I knocked on the red door. A moment later the door opened, and the kind, smiling face of a Chinese elder looked at me with inquiring eyes. "Are you Mr. Liu?" I asked, again in my best English. "No!" came the unexpected reply from the still-smiling Chinese elder with the kind face and inquiring eyes.

Not knowing what else to do or say, I pointed to the address on the paper in my hand, and the smiling Chinese elder with the ever-so-kind face and impish, inquiring eyes looked at it and said, in his best English, "Are you Danny?" "Yes!" I exclaimed and, to my great relief, he motioned me inside.

I found that behind the red door, and surrounded by the wall, was an old Japanese-style house (Taiwan had been a colony of Japan from 1895 to 1945) that looked as if it had been built sometime in the late Meiji era, but probably wasn't more than fifty years old. The Chinese elder who had so graciously let me inside ignored me completely and began tending to the various plants and flowers in the small and narrow courtyard, obviously being the gardener for Mr. Liu's family.

So, I waited for Mr. Liu to come out of his house, fully expecting him to resemble Professor Zheng in his Chinese robes, or perhaps Master Kan ("Snatch the pebble from my hand") or Master Po ("What do your hear, Grasshopper?").

A minute or so passed, and Mr. Liu was still a no-show when the red door opened behind me and another foreigner entered, greeted the gardener in Chinese, and introduced himself to me.

I told him I had just arrived in Taibei, was here to study with Mr. Liu, and was wondering when he would come out of his house to start class. My new friend just grinned, pointed to the gardener, and gently said, "He is Mr. Liu."

"The gardener is Mr. Liu?"

Before I could continue to verbally express my complete sense of disappointment ("Isn't he supposed to be wearing robes or something?"), the red door opened again, and several Chinese and another foreigner entered and also greeted the gardener with sincere respect.

Then I was somewhat more convinced that the gardener was probably Mr. Liu (especially when he called the class together). He introduced me to my new Chinese classmates and asked me, translated through the new foreign classmate who had just entered, if I would show the form I had learned.

By 1981 I had been seriously studying taiji for two years and figured I knew enough not to completely embarrass my teacher in the US, so I proceeded to do the thirty-seven-posture form of Professor Zheng Manqing.

After I had finished and was feeling rather proud of my "performance," Mr. Liu's first comment was, "Not bad." But then came the gentle admonitions. "However, you need to turn your waist. Don't use your arms independently of your body. Keep the body upright. Don't lean. Move the body as one unit."

Readers who are familiar with taiji will see that these are simply fundamental principles I had neglected to incorporate into my performance of the form. Indeed, I was to learn from Mr. Liu over the next several years not only how to incorporate these principles into the form, but also the importance of internalizing them so that, even in our daily activities, we would also naturally utilize and rely upon the taiji principles.

Despite the glaring deficiencies in my form that day, Mr. Liu never once made me feel embarrassed or inadequate, but rather he revealed to me what he essentially was in his own being: a sincere, caring, and genuinely kind teacher. This first impression I had of him never changed in the twenty-eight years I knew him.

In 1983 Mr. and Mrs. Robert W. Smith visited Mr. Liu for a few days, and I was asked to accompany them around Taibei. After their final meeting, Mr. Smith wrote quite a few notes in a pocket notebook he had, and he shared with me some of what he had written. One particular phrase Mr. Smith used in describing Mr. Liu was "the epitome of taiji." I couldn't agree more!

Indeed, Mr. Liu exemplified the taiji he had learned from Professor Zheng. He was completely unpretentious, utterly simple, and natural in his daily life, and he avoided any publicity as a taiji "master," although he truly was one by anyone's measure.

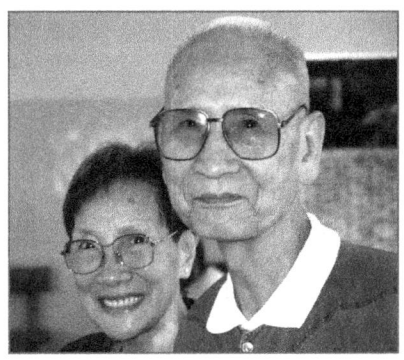

Photo of Mr. and Mrs. Liu
by Danny Emerick.

In teaching us push-hands, he emphasized the idea that in our practice we should only concentrate on "feeling" and completely eschew any notion of using the slightest force to push or to resist being pushed. "Don't be against!" (*Bu ding!*) he would admonish us, almost on a daily basis.

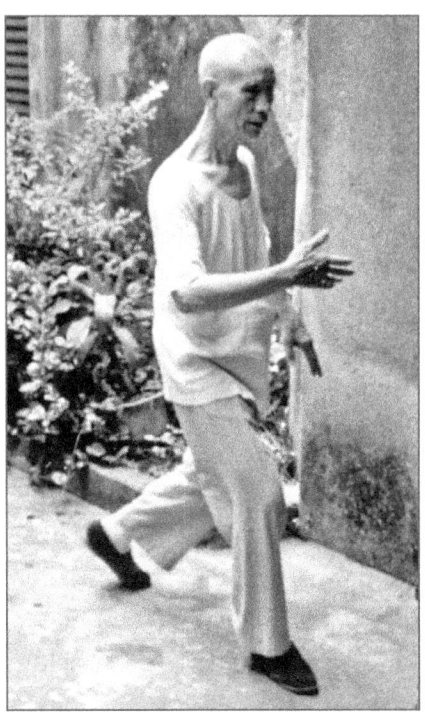

Liu Xiheng in walking ward-off.
Photo courtesy of Yuan Weiming.

Some other nuggets from Mr. Liu gleaned from class notes include the following:

- I teach the formless form.
- Taiji is simple, but not easy.
- Have a slight, light touch.
- Learn the simple; don't learn the complex.
- Pushing hands is not pushing hands . . . it is "pushing waist" [*tui yao*].
- The hand and body are like a snake, curling and curving and yielding at the slightest touch.
- Study the little curves in the form; they are the most important.
- Don't think of pushing; think only of yielding.
- Taijiquan is *keqiquan*. [*Keqi* means "manners" or "being polite"]
- Yield first!
- Everything comes from the root.
- Remember only two things: straight and relaxed. It is very simple.

And perhaps my favorite piece of advice of all the things I heard Mr. Liu say was in response to a question from my friend and classmate, Russ Mason, when we returned to Taiwan to visit Mr. Liu together in 2006. Russ asked Mr. Liu, "What taiji principles should we use to foster and improve our married life?"

Mr. Liu immediately responded by quoting a phrase in the *Taiji Classics*, "Bu ding, bu diu." Don't resist, and don't let go.

I began this brief memorial to Mr. Liu by telling how I literally mistook him for the gardener. Yet, upon further reflection, I think that he was indeed a "gardener." He never had more than a handful of students at a time, but the ones he had he tended with gentleness and care. He was always attentive to our health and well-being, and he nourished us daily with his words and by his example. This not only improved our understanding of taiji, but it also had a profound effect on our lives.

Mr. Liu has grand-students all over the world now, the result of that "garden" of students he cultivated and tended with sincere care and concern and, most importantly, with love.

May his garden continue to thrive and flourish.

(End of Danny Emerick's article)

Liu Xiheng's Western Disciples

Mr. Liu had scores of students and shared his knowledge with all. His only expectation was that a student should be "sincere" in his study with the teacher. A few wanted to show their complete sincerity to Mr. Liu and his teachings by becoming official students in the discipleship ceremony called bai shi. From 1982 until 2004, Mr. Liu accepted twenty-five disciples. Below is the list of Mr. Liu's Western disciples and the year of their bai shi:

- 1982: Mark Lord, Rick Halstead, Mike Moran, Danny Emerick
- 1984: Michael Schnapp, Bill Tucker
- 1986: Lin Farley
- 2004: Alex Makapa, Daniel Altschuler

People Mentioned in the Article

Chen Youyi	陳釉藝
Fu Kunhe	傅崑鶴
Hong Yi	弘一
Ju Hongbin	鞠鴻賓
Ke Qihua	柯啟華
Li Shutong	李叔同
Liang Tongcai	梁棟材
Liu Xiheng	劉錫亨
Luo Bangzhen	羅邦楨
Ruan Weiming	阮偉明
Shengyan	聖嚴
Su Shaoqing	蘇紹卿
Tao Bingxiang	陶炳祥
Wu Tu'nan	吳图南
Xu Yizhong	徐憶中
Xu Zhengmei	徐正梅
Yang Chengfu	楊澄甫
Ye Xiuting	葉秀挺
Yin Qitang	殷啟堂
Zhang Baokang	張寶康
Zheng Manqing	鄭曼青
Zhuangzi	莊子

Places and Terms

dantian	丹田
fashi	法師
keqi	客氣
Nanputuosi	南普陀寺
Nantou	南投
qi	氣
Raoping Xian	饒平縣
Shizhong Xue She	时中學社
taiji jian	太極劍
ting jin	聽勁
taijiquan	太極拳
tuishou	推手
wude	武德
Xiamen (Amoy)	廈門
Xindian	新店
Xuzhou	徐州
yi	意
Yonghe City	永和市
zhang men ren	掌門人
Zheng Manqing Jinian Guan	鄭曼青 紀念 館
zhong ding	中定
Zhongshan Tang (Hall)	中山堂
Zhong Xing Xin Cun	興新村

Acknowledgements

The compiler of this article wishes to thank all those who contributed to this project in ways large and small. Professor Yuan Weiming initiated the effort with his request that the Chinese source materials be translated and published for the English-speaking taijiquan community. A bow of deep gratitude is in order to Master Liu Xiheng and to the authors, Benjamin Lo, Xu Yizhong, Yuan Weiming, Xu Zhengmei, and Danny Emerick, as well as to the publishers of the *Tai Chi Journal*, in Kaohsiung, Taiwan. Yuan Weiming and Danny Emerick provided photos and other invaluable assistance, as did Robert W. Smith, Monica Chen, Warren Conner, Barbara Davis, Lin Farley, Rick Garcia, Jeff Herrod, Mark Lord, Michael Schnapp, Mark Westcott, Carol Yamasaki, and others. A special word of thanks is due Nick Tan (Chen Yuexin) and Professor Maria Tu (Du Zhongmin) for their work with the translation of source materials. Any errors are the responsibility of the compiler, and readers' corrections would be welcomed. This article is dedicated to the memory and spirit of Liu Laoshi and to his devoted family members, classmates, disciples, and students.

Bibliography

Biondi, M. (2006). Interview with grand master Hsu Yee Chung. Published on the Shizhong Study Society webpage at www.37taichi.org.tw

Cheng, M. (1962). *T'ai chi ch'uan: A simplified method of calisthenics for health and self defense.* Taibei: Shizhong Taijiquan Center.

Cheng, M. (1965/1999). *Master Cheng's new method of taichi ch'uan self-cultivation* (M. Hennessy, Trans.). Berkeley, CA: Frog, Ltd.

Cheng, M., & Smith, R. (1967/2004). *T'ai chi.* Rutland, VT: Charles E. Tuttle.

Cheng, M. (1950/1985). *Cheng Tzu's thirteen treatises on t'ai chi ch'uan* (B. Lo & M. Inn, Trans.). Richmond, CA: North Atlantic Books.

Cheng, M. (1996). *T'ai chi ch'uan: A simplified method of calisthenics for health and self defense.* [Video]. Ashville, NC: Cho San.

Chengtu Tai-Chi Chuan Research Association (2007). *Zheng Manqing Jinian Guan donors' record.* Taibei, Taiwan.

Davis, B. (1996). In search of a unified Dao: Zheng Manqing's life and contributions to taijiquan. *Journal of Asian martial arts,* 5(2), 36–59.

Davis, D., & Mann, L. (1996). Conservator of the *Taiji classics*: An interview with Benjamin Pang Jeng Lo. *Journal of Asian martial arts,* 5(4), 46–67.

Farley, L. (1986). Master Liu Hsi-Heung: We must learn to be tender, soft, and peaceful. *Free China journal,* 3(25). Reprinted in November of the same year in *Full Circle,* 1(4), 22–23.

Lo, B., Inn, M., Amacker, R., & Foe, S. (1979). *The essence of t'ai chi ch'uan: The literary tradition*. Richmond, CA: North Atlantic Books.

Liu, X. (1985). The concept of central equilibrium in taijiquan. (R. Halstead, Trans.) *T'ai chi player*, 3, 7–10.

Liu, X. (1985/2002). The concept of central equilibrium in taijiquan. (R. Halstead, Trans.) *Taijiquan journal*, 3(3), 19–23.

Mason, R. (2001). Fifty years in the fighting arts: An interview with Robert W. Smith. *Journal of Asian martial arts*, 10(1), 36–73.

Mason, R. (2008). Zheng Manqing: The memorial hall and legacy of the Master of Five Excellences in Taiwan. *Journal of Asian martial arts*, 17(3), 22–39.

Smith, R. (1974/1990). *Chinese boxing: Masters and methods*. Berkeley, CA: North Atlantic Books.

Smith, R. (1975). A master passes: A tribute to Cheng Man-ch'ing. *Shr Jung newsletter*, 1(1), 2–7.

Smith, R. (1995). Remembering Zheng Manqing: Some sketches from his life. *Journal of Asian martial arts*, 4(3), 46–59.

Smith, R. (1999). *Martial musings: A portrayal of martial arts in the 20th century*. Erie, PA: Via Media Publishing.

Tucker, W. (2008). Liu Hsi-heng: A man of principles. *T'ai chi magazine*, 32(4), 24–30.

Wile, D. (1985). *Cheng Man-Ch'ing's advanced t'ai-chi form instructions*. Brooklyn, NY: Sweet Ch'i Press.

Wile, D. (2007). *Zheng Manqing's uncollected writings on taijiquan, qigong, and health, with new biographical notes*. Milwaukee, WI: Sweet Ch'i Press.

Yang, C. (1934/2005). *Yang Chengfu: The essence and applications of taijiquan* (L. Swaim, Trans.). Berkeley, CA: North Atlantic Books.

Yang, J. (2001). *Tai chi secrets of the Yang style*. Boston, MA: YMAA Publication Center.

Yang, Z. (1988). *Yang style taijiquan*. Hong Kong: Hai Feng Publishing Co. and Beijing, China: Morning Glory Press.

Yang, Z. (1993). *Yang Chengfu shi tai ji quan*. Guangxi Province, China: Guangxi Minzu.

Yu, W., & Sharp, G. (1993 April). Fu Zhongwen: A Yang family legend. *Inside kung-fu*, 44–46.

Conservator of the *Taiji Classics*: An Interview with Benjamin Pangjeng Lo[1]
by Donald D. Davis, Ph.D. & Lawrence L. Mann*

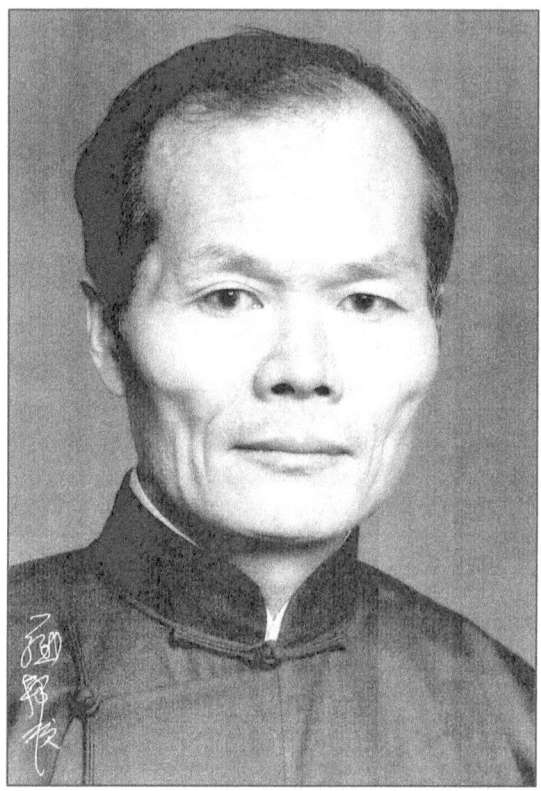

Photo courtesy of Michael Jang.

Taijiquan is one of the most famous and widely studied of the Chinese arts devoted to health, self-defense, and internal development. Its origin is uncertain, due to centuries of reliance upon oral transmission of its principles and traditions. Legend points to Zhang Sanfeng, a Daoist monk who lived in the Wudang Mountains of Hubei Province, as the founder of taijiquan.[2] Zhang allegedly lived during the Yuan dynasty (1271–1368), established by the great khans from Mongolia, although the dates of his birth and death are uncertain. Zhang reportedly combined martial movements based upon those of the snake and white crane with internal exercises derived from his Daoist practice (Yang, 1982b: 10). Taijiquan continues to distinguish itself from other martial arts by its emphasis on softness, internal development, and other Daoist principles.

Today there are many styles of taijiquan. Despite questions concerning its origins, Chen Xing traces the practice of modern styles of taijiquan to the Chen family, in China's Henan Province (Chen, 1919–1964). The style taught by Yang Luchan (1799–1872), a student of Chen Zhangxing (1771–1853), and now known simply as the Yang style is arguably the most popular style of taijiquan practiced today in the United States, probably due, at least in part, to its being the first style introduced in this country (DeMarco, 1992).

Taijiquan, with its centuries-old history, has had many distinguished teachers. Some, such as Chen Zhangxing, have enhanced the development of taijiquan through their innovation and systemization of principles and practices. Others, such as Yang Luchan and his two sons, Yang Jianhou and Yang Banhou, are famous for their martial skills. Yet others, such as Yang Chengfu, are celebrated as great proponents of the art. Still others, such as Zheng Manqing, are noted for their mastery of collateral cultural arts, such as poetry and painting, in addition to their mastery of taijiquan. Benjamin Pangjeng Lo, one of Zheng Manqing's senior students, continues this tradition.

Mr. Lo was born in April, 1927, in Jiangsu Province, China. He left with his parents for Taiwan in 1948. Mr. Lo graduated in 1953 from National Taiwan University with a bachelor's degree in Chinese literature. After graduation, he passed the civil service examination and began working for the Taiwan Provincial Government. He received a master's degree in public administration from National Chengchi University in 1968. Mr. Lo began his study of taijiquan with Zheng Manqing in 1949. He was Professor Zheng's first student in Taiwan.

Mr. Lo moved to San Francisco in 1974, where he began to teach taijiquan. Together with other students of Professor Zheng in America, he began to popularize the practice of Professor Zheng's simplified thirty-seven-posture version of the Yang form. Mr. Lo is currently retired from teaching in his San Francisco school, although he regularly conducts workshops throughout the United States, Israel, and European countries, such as Belgium, Holland, Norway, and Sweden. Looking back upon his career, Mr. Lo believes that, in addition to his teaching, his most important contributions to the spread of taijiquan have been his translation of Zheng Manqing's *Thirteen Treatises on T'ai Chi Ch'uan* (with Martin Inn), Chen Weiming's *Questions and Answers on T'ai Chi Ch'uan* (with Robert W. Smith), and his editing and translation of the *Taiji Classics: The Essence of T'ai Chi Ch'uan* (with Martin Inn, Robert Amacker, and Susan Foe). Mr. Lo's contributions to taijiquan are recognized in the Ben Lo Cup, awarded to grand champions at the annual A Taste of China, USA All-Taijiquan Championships.[3]

In this article we discuss Mr. Lo's beliefs concerning the history of taijiquan, his experiences studying with Zheng Manqing and his ideas concerning Zheng's shortened version of the Yang traditional form, his teaching experiences, philosophy, and methods, and his advice to teachers and students of taijiquan.[4] This is the first time Mr. Lo has shared these views for publication.

INTERVIEW

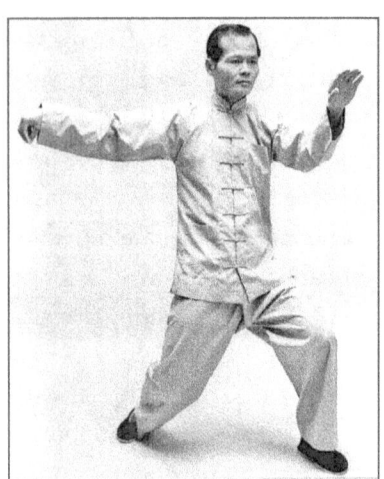
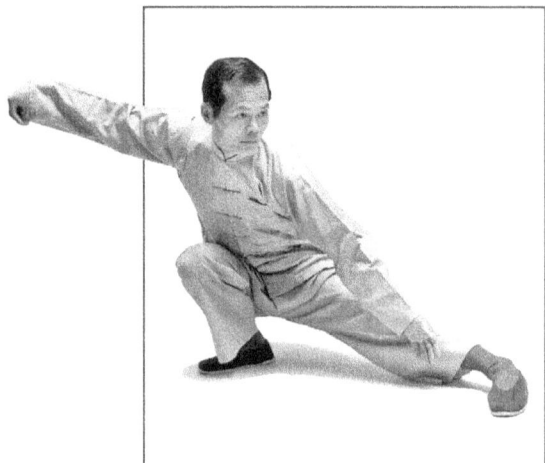

On the Origins of Taijiquan

■ Taijiquan skills provided economic and other benefits to the families and clans that possessed this knowledge. This knowledge was transmitted orally to others to maintain secrecy and because of the limited literacy of most Chinese martial artists at the time. As a result, there are few written records concerning the history of taijiquan, particularly its early years. We asked Mr. Lo to give us his thoughts concerning the origin of taijiquan.

▶ Some say Zhang Sanfeng; some even say Laozi. These are just stories handed down. There is no evidence because all of the martial arts were secret at that time. We really don't know the origin of taiji. We have to wait for the evidence. Perhaps someday some archaeologist will discover artifacts to show the early history of taijiquan. Then we will know for sure.

Today in China, some believe that the Chen family created taijiquan. How can Chen be the inventor? Some, for example Wu Tunan, even say that the Chen style is not taijiquan [Wu, 1984]. In the beginning, the Yang family called their style *mianquan* [cotton fist]. That's because it was a soft style. That's taijiquan. The Chen family called their style *paochui* [strike like a cannon]. Also, the Chen family doesn't have the *Taiji Classics*.[5] The *Taiji Classics* are like the taiji bible. Some of the most important principles from the *Taiji Classics* are relax, separate yin and yang, make the waist the commander, keep the body upright and movements slow. The Chen style doesn't adhere to these principles. Later, when Yang Luchan became famous, the Chen family called their style taijiquan. All styles of taijiquan—Chen, Yang, both Wu styles, Sun, and so forth—should follow the principles described in the *Taiji Classics* if they are going to call themselves taijiquan. If the Chen family invented taiji, why don't they have the *Taiji Classics*?[6]

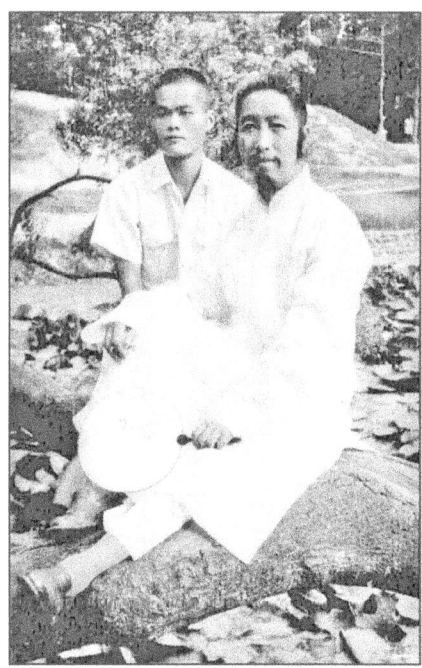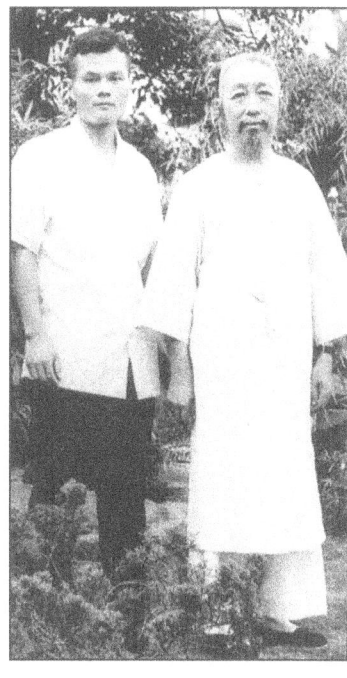

Photographs of Benjamin Lo with Zheng Manqing
taken in Taibei, Taiwan.
Photo courtesy of Benjamin Lo.

■ Huang (1979: 61–62) states that Yang Luchan, after studying with the Chen family, probably returned to the original concepts of Zhang Sanfeng and Wang Zongyue to create a new school that took his name. That is, Yang may have changed the style of taijiquan that he learned from the Chen family in order to emphasize these earlier principles.[7]

▶ I think that this is an inference based on incomplete information. I do not believe there is any evidence to support Huang's claim. At this point, no one knows for certain from whom Yang Luchan received the taiji principles. Yang may have received these principles from Chen Zhangxing and Wu Yuxiang.

On the Origins of Taijiquan

I first sought out Professor Zheng because I was sick and he was a famous medical doctor and friend of my father. Western-trained doctors I visited said I had neurological problems, but the Professor diagnosed my illness as an internal injury. He gave me some herb medicine to take and suggested I begin to practice taiji to make my body stronger so that it could absorb the medicine he was giving me. I asked him where I could study taiji, and he said I could learn from him. I looked at him and thought to myself that he was not a martial arts teacher. I asked, "You know taiji?" He said he knew a little—enough to teach me! At that time I felt surprised, because I didn't know that he was a martial arts expert. Later on, many famous martial artists came to visit him. They told me how famous he was, but at the time I didn't know. Gradually I found out that he had been head of the martial arts school in Hunan Province. He presented himself quite simply, even to me. That's the Chinese way. After about three months, I began to improve and feel better. After I started to feel better, I became very serious about practicing taiji because it gave me hope of recovery from my illness. Before then, I'd been sick for a long time and had little hope for improvement. At this time I was twenty.

For the first four years of training, I improved rapidly. But after five years, I began to feel frustrated and I thought about quitting. I'd reached a plateau and didn't feel that I was improving. Later, I also felt like quitting after fifteen years and after twenty-six years of practice. Each time classmates would push with me and encourage me. This helped me to maintain my practice. Also, I learned to compare my practice with myself and not with others. For instance, I believed that it was a good achievement if last year I caught a cold, but this year I didn't catch one. Throughout this time, I studied only with Professor Zheng. I have never been able to master everything he taught to me, so it never seemed sensible to me to study other martial arts or with other teachers.

■ Zheng Manqing began his martial arts training as a student of Yang Chengfu, grandson of Yang Luchan, founder of the Yang school of taijiquan.[8]
▶ The Professor began to study taiji because he had an advanced stage of tuberculosis [third degree] from which he thought he would not recover. After a while, he began to improve, but he quit practicing because he became too busy. Then he got sick again. He went through this cycle of practice followed by improvement and quitting practice followed by relapse twice more before deciding never to quit again.

■ Professor Zheng was an accomplished man, the Master of Five Excellences—taijiquan, painting, calligraphy, poetry, and traditional Chinese medicine. For Zheng, the common theme underlying each of these arts was his study and application of the principles of Confucianism and Daoism, and the opportunity to live in harmony with the Way. Sutton (1994) states that Professor Zheng, because of his experience in these other arts, changed his practice of the form enough to merit a new name—the Zheng style of taijiquan. Lo (1985) and Smith (1995) have rebutted this claim. Mr. Lo wished to explain.

▶ Some people say that Zheng Manqing changed the Yang form, but it's not true. What was changed? Which parts of his simplified form aren't the same as the Yang form? His major contribution to taiji was simplification of the Yang form. There is no such thing as the Zheng style of taiji. Professor Zheng could not create his form because it was already there; it was the Yang form. He explains how he shortened the Yang form and his reasons for simplifying it in his *Thirteen Treatises* (Zheng, 1950/1985). He simplified it by deleting repetitions; the longer Yang form merely repeats the parts that were extracted into the simplified form. He did this because it took too long to learn and master the long form. Today, people and their lifestyles have changed, and they don't have the patience to learn and practice the long form. Also, in the old days taiji was practiced as a serious martial art. People who practiced it were willing to commit the time required to master it. Today many people practice taiji for health and exercise. They aren't so serious and don't have the time to learn and master the long form.

When one states that teachers have changed the way they do the form, it's sometimes due to faulty perception and limited understanding of the form. This problem also occurs when teachers teach the form before they've mastered it themselves. Sometimes when a student observes others doing taiji and their postures seem different, it's the student's fault. Usually when a posture seems changed, it's because the student isn't doing the posture correctly; he isn't following the principles. Even now, when I ask students . . . to do the postures, they can't do them; they can't maintain the taiji principles while doing these postures. If those students teach someday, their students will follow them in doing the postures incorrectly. Then the posture will appear to be changed. The Professor's classmate, Chen Weiming, was asked by his students, "Why does each teacher do the form differently?" Chen answered, "Students change the postures because they did not learn them correctly in the first place." Also, in the old days teachers were very strict; a student wouldn't dare ask a question if he didn't understand what the teacher taught him.[9]

The Professor simplified the form during the Sino-Japanese War.[10] He was in charge of martial arts training in Hunan Province. Martial arts instructors from throughout the province came to be trained by him. After discovering that there wasn't enough time to teach the long form to those who wanted to learn taiji, the Professor shortened the form. He didn't simplify the form with the intention of increasing its popularity, as some people believe. No, he didn't have this ambition when he simplified the form. He merely thought that more people would be willing to invest the time to learn taiji if it didn't take so long to do. Later on, it just happened to become popular.

■ Professor Zheng must have been an extraordinary person with great confidence in his own ability to simplify the form taught to him by Yang Chengfu.
▶ Yes, he was a very special person. At the age of eighteen most people are in high school, but he was already a professor in a university.[11] How many people are expert at painting, Chinese medicine, calligraphy, and poetry in addition to taiji? Around the age of thirty he was president of the National Association for Practitioners of Traditional Chinese Medicine. Every city and province in China had an association and president, yet he became leader of them all at quite a young age. At the same time, he was president of a fine arts college.[12] People followed him because of his achievements. He had exceptional natural gifts as a human being.

■ We were astonished to learn that, during twenty-six years of studying with Professor Zheng Manqing, Mr. Lo never saw him do the form in its entirety during practice or instruction.
▶ The only chance I had to see the Professor do the form was when some organization invited him to give a speech and the audience asked him to do the form. Then he would do the whole thing. But I never saw him do it by himself. Nobody saw that. It's like, if you study singing with Pavarotti, you wouldn't say to him: "Please sing this part for me. Let me see how you sing it." When he taught me, he taught me one posture at a time. First this part, then the next part, and so forth. When I began to study taiji forty-eight years ago, I remember that going from single whip to lifting hands took 120 hours.[13] At this time, Mrs. Zheng observed me doing the form. She was surprised that I hadn't learned more postures. She asked the Professor why he hadn't taught me more, and he said that my leg was shaking like a *pipa* string.[14] She said that times change, and the Professor shouldn't teach me like Grandmaster Yang taught him. After this, the Professor began to teach me the next postures. Later, he changed his teaching style when he came to the United States. In fact, I was surprised to learn when I visited the Professor's New York school that the students there had seen him do the entire form.

Professor Zheng taught students in China differently from the way he taught students in the United States. When he taught me, he was very strict, especially when he was younger. My legs would be so sore that, when I went to bed at night,

I had to use my hands to lift my legs onto the bed. He was kinder with American students. He got softer as he grew older. The Professor also said in the *Thirteen Treatises* that practicing taiji made him softer.

■ Zheng Manqing did not practice with weapons often used by Yang style practitioners—for example, broadsword, spear, and staff—although he greatly enjoyed practicing the taiji straight sword.

▶ I know he learned the sword and spear. He really enjoyed the sword. He showed me how to use the spear once in his study. I don't know why he did not use these other weapons. Perhaps Master Yang didn't have time to teach him, or maybe Professor Zheng didn't have time to learn. At that time, when Professor Zheng was twenty-eight or thirty, he was president of a fine arts college; maybe he was too busy.

Professor Zheng wanted to teach me the sword, but I told him I didn't want to learn it. I had trained hard but couldn't do the form perfectly yet, so why waste time on learning the sword?

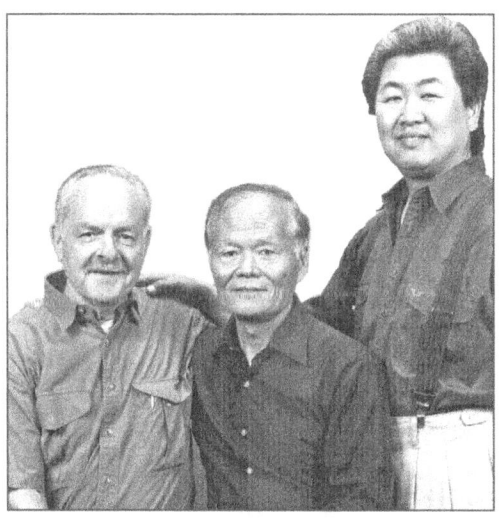

Left to right: Robert W. Smith, Benjamin Lo, and Patrick Cheng, Professor Zheng's son. Photo courtesy of Tim Barnwell.

■ Despite his early resistance, after practicing the taiji form for fifteen years, Mr. Lo learned the sword form at Professor Zheng's insistence. Since coming to the United States, Mr. Lo has taught the sword form only twice to a small group of selected students who already had a good foundation in the taiji form. He also recognized that students in the United States wished to learn more quickly and were not prepared to wait as long as he to learn the sword form.

"No burn, no earn; no pain, no gain."
—Benjamin Lo

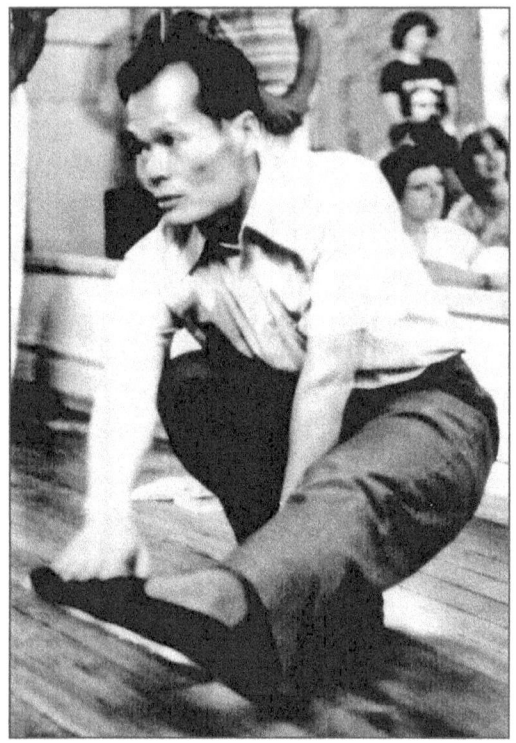

Benjamin Lo in a variation of
snake creeps down, also known
as squatting single whip.
Note that Mr. Lo is utterly relaxed
and picking up his front foot.
Photo courtesy of R. W. Smith.

Teaching, Philosophy, and Methods

■ Benjamin Lo is a traditionalist. His teaching emphasizes the *Taiji Classics* and the proper practice of each posture in Zheng Manqing's simplified version of the Yang form. He teaches in the same manner in which he was taught. Mr. Lo is noted for asking his students to stand still and to sink low in each posture. He often tells students, "Remember my name—'bend low'" (Ben Lo), to encourage strengthening each posture. We asked Mr. Lo to share advice he would give to students and teachers of taijiquan.

▶ If a person really wants to learn taiji, he should look for a teacher who follows the principles described in the *Taiji Classics*—for example, relax, separate yin and yang, sink the qi, keep the body upright, and so forth.[15] If the teacher doesn't follow the principles, do you think this is taiji? Real taiji has to follow the principles described in the *Taiji Classics*.

You must practice the form every day, morning and night, and hold the postures. You need to hold the postures to get stronger. To get good, you need to *chikou* [literally, "to eat bitter," meaning to work very hard despite difficulties]. That's why I say, the more you suffer, the more you gain. It's like depositing money in the bank. You can't put one penny in the bank and get a lot of interest. If you put more money in the bank, you'll get more interest. I always tell my students, "No burn, no earn; no pain, no gain." But to avoid injury, you shouldn't overdo it.

To be good, a taiji player requires several things: natural gifts, proper attitude, perseverance, and a good teacher. One natural gift is the ability to comprehend the *Taiji Classics*. This is a type of taiji intelligence. With some people, you explain something a hundred times and they still don't get it. With others, you explain it once and they understand. It's like the bell curve, where most people have average intelligence, and a small number are more intelligent than average, and another small number are less intelligent than average. Some people just comprehend the principles of taiji more easily.

Another natural gift is the ability to relax the body. If you can't relax, taiji doesn't work. Like gymnastics or swimming, where physical gifts provide advantage, some people are more capable of relaxing and therefore of excelling in taiji.

Proper attitude is the second thing required to be skilled in taiji. Attitude refers to whether you are serious about your practice.

Perseverance is the third quality needed for success in taiji. If you have great natural ability but lack perseverance, you can't become very good.

Finally, you need a good teacher. Without a good teacher, you can't learn the proper way to do taiji. A good teacher is like having a compass when you're in the jungle. The compass shows you the correct path to take. Without a good teacher, you can't find the right way to practice.

■ Besides doing the form, Mr. Lo stresses the practice of push-hands (tuishou) to learn the application of taiji principles. In push-hands, the postures from the form are practiced with a partner. The purpose of push-hands is to learn to sense and control a partner's energy. One should learn to be as sensitive as the "feelers of a cricket" (Wang & Zheng, 1983: 188). The ability to sense and control a partner's energy is required to master taijiquan.

▶ In pushing hands we learn feeling. Professor Zheng always said, "Know yourself through practicing the form; know others through practicing pushing hands."[16] Through pushing hands, you can tell something about a person's character, for example, whether they're gentle or aggressive. Pushing hands teaches sticking to your partner. In taiji we stay close to the joints, for example, the wrists, elbows and shoulders. In some ways this sticking is like *qinna*, but it's also different.[17] In qinna, you stay close to your partner's joints like in taiji, but in taiji we use the whole body to break the partner's balance.

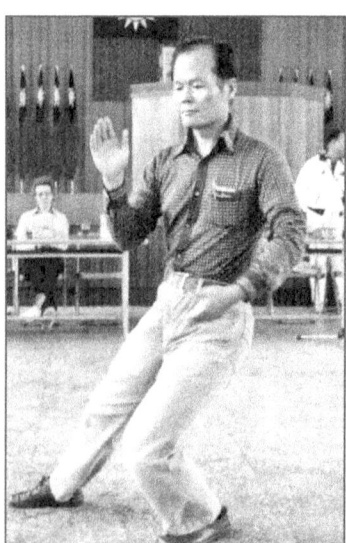 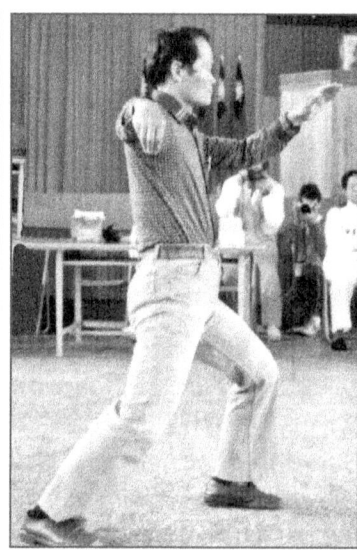 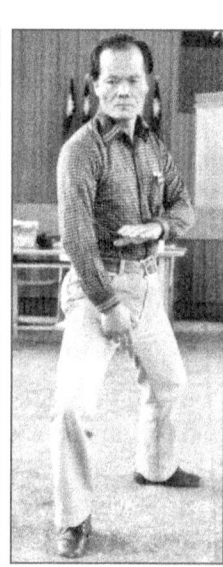

Taijiquan postures photographed
in Taiwan: rollback, single whip,
and shoulder stroke.
Courtesy of Robert W. Smith.

■ Lowenthal (1994: 63) states that one must be aware of three points of contact when practicing push-hands: the partner's two elbows and leading wrist. It is through these three points, he writes, that one senses and controls the partner's energy. Mr. Lo expands on this idea.

▶ The Professor said, "The whole body is a hand and the hand is not a hand." This means the whole body should act at one time. The Professor wrote that he once dreamed that he had no arms, and after awakening he finally understood how to move in taiji. In other words, when doing push-hands one must use the entire body, not just the arms and hands, to sense one's partner and move in response to his actions.

■ Practicing applications and push-hands is required to learn the martial arts aspects of taiji.

▶ The study of martial arts is hard work. Most people can't take it. I always tell people that, although the Hong Kong gongfu movies exaggerate the difficulty of training, they're partly true. You have to work really hard. Holding the postures is important, but you must be relaxed. Your body can't be stiff as a rock. For example, when I teach classes, I tell people to assume a posture and not move, but after one or two minutes they stand up and move around. This isn't the way to excel in the martial arts.

When the Professor taught push-hands, he said that when you touch people, in one second it should be like a clock—tick, you touch me; tock, you're out. You learn this through practicing push-hands (tuishou). But if your form is no good, you can't do anything in push-hands. If you have time, you can learn pushing hands; if you don't have time, you don't have to learn it, especially if you just do the form for exercise.

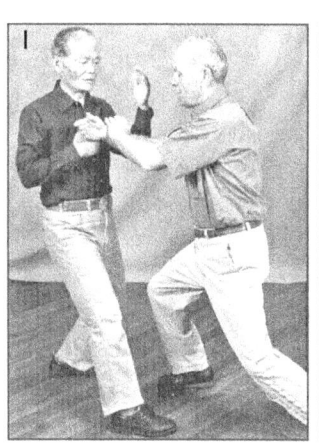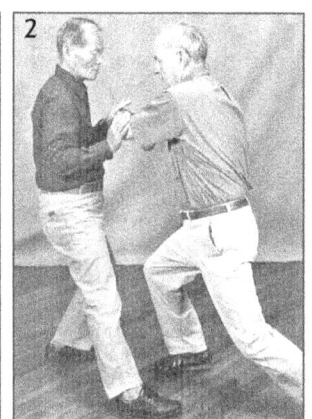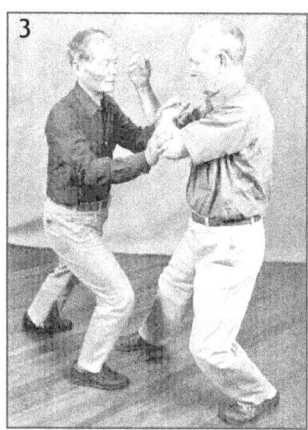

Mr. Lo and R. W. Smith pushing hands.
1) When Lo neutralizes Smith's push with rollback, Smith changes to press.
2) Lo neutralizes Smith's press and begins to push.
3) Smith uses rollback to neutralize.
Photographs courtesy of R. W. Smith.

■ Bagua and xingyi are the internal cousins of taijiquan (Smith, 1981a, 1981b). We asked Mr. Lo if studying these or other arts would help one to master taiji.

▶ You think Yang Luchan learned bagua or xingyi? You think Dong Haichuan, founder of bagua, learned taiji? Do you think Li Cunyi, a great master of xingyi, studied bagua or taiji? No! If you cannot be good at one thing, how can you learn other things? However, bagua, xingyi and taiji do share certain principles derived from the *Book of Changes* [*Yijing*], and they all rely on yin and yang.

■ Given taijiquan's historical foundation in Daoism and the fact that throughout his lifetime Zheng Manqing and studied the *Yijing* and *Daodejing* (Zheng, 1950/1985, 1981), we asked whether study of these classical texts is necessary for the mastery of taiji.

▶ No, no, not at all. If this were necessary, university professors who teach about the *Yijing* would also be taiji masters. Also, some taiji masters, such as Yang Chengfu, were not highly educated. His reputation was strong because his taiji was good. Of course, it's not bad if you read these books, but it's not enough. Other books like Sunzi's are also useful.[18] But we have to know the difference between Daoist philosophy and Daoist religion. Taiji is related to Daoist philosophy but not to Daoist religion. Elements of Daoist philosophy—yin and yang, five elements theory, practices to extend longevity—have something to do with taiji. However, the student of taiji must be careful that he doesn't just study books, that he not become a mere armchair boxer.

The mind is important in taiji. For example, if I tell you to move your hand here, you can do that. Now if I tell you to put your mind [yi] here, what does that mean? It means you have to direct your attention and focus to this spot. If you can't do this, you can't do anything. But you can't force it. You go naturally, little by little. First, direct your mind for a short time, then for a longer time. The way you learn to do this is by practicing the form. When you start to learn the form, of course, you think about each posture. Gradually with practice, you can think about other things because you no longer have to concentrate on doing the postures. But later, after you master the form, you just do it. You forget yourself. You forget everything. You just do the form. It's like going to visit some pretty place. You don't pay attention to any one thing in particular. What's pretty? All of it together is pretty.

■ Related to the use of mind to direct actions is the difference between li (force) and jin (internal strength) as sources of power in taijiquan.

▶ Li is derived from the bones, while jin is derived from the ligaments. Li is used by moving in a straight line, while jin is used by moving in a curve. Jin is also related to the development of the qi and is more powerful than li. That's why in push-hands we try to use jin to neutralize a partner's force. You relax, stick to him, and neutralize him when he pushes you—that's jin. But the form is important too. Without the form, you can't develop jin. Practicing the form is like putting money into the bank. When you get more money, then you can spend some (jin). However, a lot of people have money, but they don't know how to use it properly. That's the use of jin too. That's why we have to practice push-hands, to learn how to use jin.

■ We asked Mr. Lo to describe the relationship among taijiquan, qigong, and other forms of internal strength training.[19] We first asked if Professor Zheng had ever studied internal strength training with Zuo Laipeng, as stated by Sutton (1994).[20]

▶ The Professor never received any internal strength training from Zuo Laipeng. The Professor never learned any Zuo style of taiji. The only thing the Professor practiced throughout his life other than the Yang form was *yijin* [muscle/tendon changing]. When he got older, around sixty, he also began to meditate. He did taiji meditation by just sitting and sinking the qi into the dantian.[21] In taiji meditation you don't need to count the breaths or breathe in any special way. When you practice taiji, you gradually learn how to breathe naturally.

When people do qigong, they repeat one posture. Taiji has a variety of qigong postures. To me, any part of taiji is qigong. So if people do taiji, they also do qigong. Taiji is a form of *neijiaquan* [internal art]; it develops the qi. Now if you have time, you can learn other methods of qigong. They are not in opposition to taiji principles. But if you have extra time, I feel it would be better spent on practicing taiji because taiji uses the whole body. If you are thirsty, you drink a glass of water. Should you drink orange juice too? You don't have to. Also, you can't learn everything. In China there are more than one thousand kinds of qigong. If you learn one every year, or even one every day, there isn't enough time. And you need time to practice every one.[22]

■ Some taiji teachers emphasize the use of music while practicing the form or practicing the mirror image of the form. We asked Mr. Lo to comment on these practices.

▶ The Chinese have practiced taiji for several hundred years without these things. In Confucius's time, we already had classical music. Do you think that the founder of taiji didn't know about or think about using music? As for doing the form on both sides, if you want to do it, why not? Some people are left handed, and some people are right handed. But you don't have to do it this way because in the form we already practice on both sides. Also, the founder of taiji wasn't stupid. If he thought practicing on both sides was necessary, he would have put it in the form.

■ We followed up by asking Mr. Lo if he thought the form was perfect as it is or whether it could be improved.

▶ We can't even follow it as it is. When people can't finish what they are eating, why offer them more food? What I give you, you can't even digest, and you want more? But I would never say no. Nothing is perfect. Maybe in the future somebody like Yang Luchan may improve the form, but this kind of person is very rare. We simply don't know.

■ Taiji schools experience conflict at times. This conflict sometimes exists between teacher and students or, more often, between students themselves. We asked Mr. Lo to share his thoughts regarding proper relationships among those who practice taiji.
▶ First, you should respect your teacher. That's ethical. I feel very strongly about this. Even if I learn more and become better than my teacher, he is still my teacher. Without him, I wouldn't know taiji at all. However, if I'm the teacher and you've learned everything I know, then I'd tell you I have nothing more to teach you and then tell you where to go next to study. I would write a letter to introduce you to a new teacher, to recommend you as a good person. This other teacher may then accept you as his student. But you shouldn't sneak to work with this other teacher. That's not right. You have to tell your teacher if you plan to study with someone else. I've refused some students who wanted to work with me. They came from Taiwan, where they were the students of teachers I knew there. I asked for their letter of introduction, but they didn't have one. I knew that they were sneaking to study with me. If they do this now to their teacher, someday they'll do it to me too. It's not honest.

The number 1 student is the one who has trained with the teacher the longest. If the teacher retires, he usually leaves the school to the number 1 student. But this is not always the best student. Sometimes, a younger student may have more natural ability. If the number 1 student is not the best, then he knows that he will cause the school to lose face, so he may ask the best student to take charge. But this younger student will still have to respect and listen to his senior classmate. This requires good character. But the teacher knows this too. I wouldn't want my school ruined by leaving in charge a student who didn't have good character and a high level of skill.

■ Traditionally, Chinese martial arts teachers are reputed to keep the secrets of their masters until they reach the last hours before their death. Sometimes these secrets die with them. We asked Mr. Lo to share with us a secret learned from his many years of studying and teaching taijiquan.
▶ The teacher can only show you how to do it. The rest is all your work. The secret is to practice.

APPENDIX—Transliteration of Chinese Terms

Pinyin	Wade-Giles	Pinyin	Wade-Giles
bagua	pa-kua	Quanzhen sect	Ch'üan-chen sect
Chan Buddhist	Ch'an Buddhist	Sunzi	Sun-tzu (Sun-tsu)
Chen	Ch'en	taiji, taijiquan	t'ai chi, t'ai chi ch'üan
Chen Wangting	Ch'en Wang-t'ing	tuishou	t'ui-shou
Chen Weiming	Ch'en Wei-ming	waijiaquan	wai chia ch'üan
Chen Xing	Ch'en Hsing	Wang Beixing	Wang Pei-hsing
Chen Zhangxing	Ch'en Chang-hsing	Wang Maozhai	Wang Mao-chai
chikou	ch'ih-k'ou	Wang Zhengnan	Wang Cheng-nan
Damo	Ta-mo	Wang Zongyue	Wang Tsung-yüeh
dantian	tan-t'ien	Wudang Mountains	Wutang Mountains
Daodejing	*Tao Te Ch'ing*	Wu Tunan	Wu T'u-nan
Daoism, Daoist	Taoism, Taoist	Wu Guozhong	Wu Kuo-ch'ung
Dong Haichuan	Tung Hai-ch'üan	Wu Heqing	Wu Ho-ch'ing
Fu Zili	Fu Tzu-li	Wu Qiuying	Wu Ch'iu-ying
gongfu	kung-fu	Wu You	Wu Yu
Han Gongyue	Han Kung-yüeh	Wu Yuxiang	Wu Yü-hsiang
Henan Province	Honan Province	xiangyi	hsing-yi
Huang Lizhou	Huang Li-ch'ou	Xu Chen	Hsü Chen
Hubei Province	Hupei Province	Xu Xuanping	Hsü Hsüan-p'ing
Hunan Province	Hunan Province	Yang	Yang
Jiangsu Province	Chiangsu Province	Yang Banhou	Yang Pan-hou
jin	chin	Yang Chengfu	Yang Ch'eng-fu
Laozi	Lao-tzu (Lao-tsu)	Yang Jianhou	Yang Ch'ien-hou
li	li	Yang Luchan	Yang Lu-ch'an
Li Cunyi	Li Ts'un-i	Yang Yuding	Yang Yu-ting
Li Yiyu	Li Yi-yü	Yang Zhenduo	Yang Chen-tuo
mianquan	mien-ch'üan	Ye Jimei	Yeh Chi-mei
Ming	Ming	yi	i
neijiaquan	nei chia ch'üan	*Yijinjing*	*Yi Chin Ching*
Ninbo	Ningpo	*Yi Jing*	*I Ching*
Paochui	P'ao-ch'ui	Ying Lihen	Ying Li-hen
pipa	p'i-pa	Yuan	Yüan
qi	ch'i	Yuwen University	Yü-wen University
qigong	ch'i-kung	Zhang Qinling	Chang Ch'in-ling
qinna	ch'in-na	Zhang Sanfeng	Chang San-feng
Qing Dynasty	Ch'ing Dynasty	Zheng Manqing	Cheng Man-ch'ing
Quan You	Ch'üan Yu	Zuo Laipeng	Tso Lai-p'eng

* NOTE: Work on this article was assisted by a Fulbright Fellowship awarded to the first author and by resources provided by Wuhan University, in China, and the Department of Psychology at the University of Virginia, where the first author was a visiting professor.

Acknowledgements

We are grateful to Robert W. Smith for his help. His comments on earlier versions of this article reveal why he is the dean of martial arts scholars. Of course, we accept all responsibility for any remaining errors. We thank Peggy Kinard for her help in preparing transcripts of our taped interviews.

Notes

[1] Pinyin, the transliteration system employed today in China, rather than the more traditional Wade-Giles system, is used for all Chinese terms except references published using the Wade-Giles system. We retained existing Wade-Giles titles in our bibliography to make it easier for readers to locate them although we used pinyin for all authors' names to make them consistent with citations in the text. We include in the appendix Pinyin terms and their Wade-Giles equivalents. We used Wu (1979) to choose equivalent terms.

[2] Belief in Zhang Sanfeng as the founder of taijiquan is widespread, although there is little historical evidence to support this claim. Chen Weiming (1929/1985: 13) states that, according to the *Ningbo Chronicle*, Huang Lizhou wrote at the end of the Ming dynasty (1368–1644) that Wang Zhengnan's tombstone shows taijiquan was transmitted to Zhang Sanfeng and Ye Jimei. Chen also states that taiji was transmitted to four other people: Xu Xuanping, Fu Zili, Han Gongyue, and Ying Lihen.

Jou (1981: 2) states that Zhang Sanfeng was born at midnight on April 9, 1247. Lo, Inn, Amacker, and Foe (1985: 9) state that the time during which Zhang is believed to have lived is 1279–1368, although legend has it that he lived more than 250 years. Liao (1990: 10) states that Zhang founded his temple on Wudang Mountain in 1200, decades before the date Jou or Lo and his colleagues cite for his birth. Seidel (1970: 485–487) states that Zhang began his study of Daoism years after the time that Liao says he founded his first temple on Wudang Mountain and that he died around 1393. Differences in these dates demonstrate the uncertainty concerning the facts of Zhang Sanfeng's life.

Seidel (1970), in a careful historical study, provides the following conclusions. Zhang Sanfeng was a Daoist master who was loosely connected with the Quanzhen sect of Daoism, received imperial honors, and founded several retreats in the Wudang Mountains. She could discover no evidence to demonstrate that he was the founder of taijiquan. The association of taijiquan with Zhang Sanfeng seems instead to represent an attempt to add historical validity to the lineage of internal martial arts (neijiaquan), just as Damo (Bodhidharma) has been used to validate the origin of external styles (*waijiaquan*) at the Shaolin Temple.

Records concerning the history of taijiquan become more reliable during the late Ming (1368–1644) and Qing (1644–1912) dynasties. Some evidence points to Chen Wangting (1597–1644) and his family, with influence from Wang Zongyue (1736–1795), as the source of modern taijiquan styles. Seidel (1970: 505) states that Wu Heqing, a student of Yang Luchan, wrote about taijiquan, and that Wu ascribed the origin of his writings to Wang Zongyue to give them more weight. Yang Zhenduo, third son of Yang Chengfu, states that taijiquan was founded at the end of the Ming dynasty, presumably by Chen Wangting, although he does not state this explicitly (Yang, 1988: l). See DeMarco (1992) for a discussion of the origin and evolution of various taijiquan lineages.

3 Pat Rice, cofounder and director of A Taste of China, USA All-Taijiquan Championships, one of the oldest and largest taijiquan tournaments in the United States, explained why the grand champion trophy is named the Ben Lo Cup. She states that this was done to encourage competitors to maintain proper taiji principles while pushing hands. She says that, because Mr. Lo has such a high level of skill and embodies taiji principles in his practice and teaching, he serves as an exemplar for serious practitioners of the art.

4 We took Mr. Lo's responses from transcripts of interviews conducted in March and June 1995, and April 1996. We have edited his comments, and he has reviewed our editing to ensure accuracy.

5 The *Taiji Classics* are a collection of songs and poems written in classical Chinese that were used to aid in the oral transmission of taijiquan principles. Although some of the writings are alleged to be more than one thousand years old, the evidence for this is inconclusive. The facts seem to be that they were discovered in the middle of the nineteenth century in a salt shop by Wu Qiuying, who took them to his brother Wu Yuxiang (creator of the Wu style of taijiquan). Wu Yuxiang then showed the manuscript to his teacher, Yang Luchan, who interpreted them for Wu due to their being written in a form of taiji code. From this point, both Yang and Wu incorporated the *Taiji Classics* into their teaching. The compiler of the *Taiji Classics* was reputed to be Wang Zongyue, the eighteenth century visitor to the Chen family village, but this is probably not true. In addition to works allegedly written by Wang Zongyue, the *Taiji Classics* contain writings attributed to Zhang Sanfeng, Wu Yuxiang, and Li Yiyu. Moreover, modern taiji writings by Yang Chengfu and his students Chen Weiming and

Zheng Manqing were added later (see Lo et al., 1985). Still other writings were provided by anonymous authors. Liao (1990), Lo et al. (1985), and Yang (1987) provide different compilations and translations. The principles expounded in the *Taiji Classics* continue to provide the foundation for the Zheng Manqing school of taijiquan, as well as other practitioners of the Yang style.

6 Some may say the *Taiji Classics* were written by practitioners of the Yang family style. If this is true, it would be obvious that they would emphasize the Yang manner of doing the postures. The story concerning the discovery of the *Taiji Classics* manuscripts by Wu Qiuying, who took them to his brother Wu Yuxiang, a practitioner of the Yang family style, supports this claim. On the other hand, the Yang family was illiterate and incapable of writing the *Taiji Classics*. Nevertheless, allegations that the *Taiji Classics* had a more ancient origin would be more believable had they been discovered by someone outside of the Yang family circle.

7 Huang (1979: 62) cites a study of the history of taijiquan written by Xu Chen and published in Hong Kong that states that it was Yang Luchan who first attributed the origin of taijiquan to Zhang Sanfeng.

8 Sutton (1994: 58; also footnote 1) states that Professor Zheng began his martial arts training with Shaolin boxing during his youth, not with taijiquan, as we claim. He cites Zheng's biography engraved on the wall of his tomb and translated and published in English by Tam Gibbs. Mr. Lo states that this was a mistranslation by Gibbs. He states further that Zheng instead studied a set of stretching exercises associated with the *Yijinjing* (*Muscle/Tendon Changing Classic*) during his youth, not Shaolin boxing. Moreover, Jou (1981: A19), citing the preface to Zheng's 1946 book on taijiquan, says that Zheng practiced yijin to cure himself of rickets and rheumatism he suffered in his youth. Yijin, a form of qigong employing massage and Chan Buddhist and Daoist meditation practices, was allegedly created by Damo (Bodhidharma) at the Shaolin Temple and later incorporated into various forms of boxing practiced there (Yang, 1989: 11). Given its connection with the Shaolin Temple and some of its forms of boxing, Tam Gibbs apparently confused *Yijinjing* with a Shaolin style of boxing.

9 Emphasis on family transmission and the "closed door" approach to teaching contributed to the uncertainty concerning the history and teaching of taijiquan and other Chinese martial arts. As a result of this tradition of secrecy, knowledge of different styles was limited and distortions marked the knowledge that was transmitted. Moreover, the emphasis on hierarchy in Chinese society amplified the social distance between teacher and student. This distance prevented students from asking questions to seek correction of mistakes. Even today, many teachers in China feel insulted if a student asks questions because this ques-

tioning implies that the teacher did not teach the lesson clearly enough for the student to understand. Questioning also reflects on the student's character by suggesting that the student is not very adept or has not studied very hard. It is hardly surprising that errors occur and remain uncorrected within this type of learning environment. The relative openness of the Western teaching tradition and the greater tendency of Western, especially North American, students to ask questions merely make corrections and discussion of them more salient.

10 Smith (1995) states that Zheng Manqing may have been experimenting with a simplified version of the Yang form in 1938, and that it did not become finalized until 1947, just before he moved to Taiwan. Lo (1985) also states that Zheng adopted the simplified form in 1938.

11 Zheng taught at Yuwen University in Beijing. He became director of the Department of Chinese Painting at the Shanghai School of Fine Arts when in his midtwenties. See the short biography written by Tam Gibbs and printed in Zheng (1981).

12 Professor Zheng was president of the College of Chinese Culture and Arts in Shanghai, which he cofounded when in his late twenties (Zheng, 1981).

13 Single whip and lifting hands are the eighth and ninth postures in Zheng's simplified form.

14 A pipa is a Chinese plucked string instrument with a fretted fingerboard, similar to a Western lute or classical guitar.

15 "Separate yin and yang" refers to the division of weight between one's legs. According to traditional Chinese theories of human physiology and medicine, qi is the energy that travels along a network of meridians throughout the body. Development and use of the qi is a goal of advanced taiji practice.

16 Wang Beixing (a student of Yang Yuding and his teacher Wang Maozhai), who teaches the Wu style today in Beijing, states, seek "to know one's own energy through the sequence practice, and the other's energy through push-hands exercise" (Wang & Zeng, 1983: 189). Given that Wang Beixing's teacher—Wang Maozhai—was a student of Quan You (also known as Wu You), founder of the Wu style, who was in turn a student of Yang Banhou, Yang Luchan's son, this teaching concerning sensing energy is clearly part of the Yang-style tradition. It is, therefore, obvious that Zheng Manqing should continue to impart this insight to his students, demonstrating his root in the Yang tradition.

17 Qinna emphasizes striking nerves and manipulation of muscles, fascia, and joints to subdue one's opponent. It is generally associated with external martial arts (waijiaquan) (see Smith, 1996; Yang, 1982a).

18 Sunzi is the author of the *The Art of War* (Sun, 1988), an ancient treatise devoted to military strategy that is still studied widely throughout Asia.

[19] Qigong is a system of deep-breathing exercises that have associated physical movements. The Chinese have practiced qigong for many centuries to improve health and increase longevity. Qigong is very popular today in China, more popular than taijiquan, with many instructional programs broadcast on television and published in the popular press.

[20] Sutton (1994) claims that Zheng Manqing studied internal strength techniques under Zuo Laipeng. He cites Wu Guozhong (1985) to support his claim. Lo (1985) and Smith (1995) demonstrate why this claim is false. Lo (1985) states further that there is no such thing as a Zuo style of taijiquan. Zheng really learned a method of internal energy cultivation from Zhang Qinlin, a senior classmate who studied with Zuo Laipeng.

[21] The dantian is a point in the abdomen about 1.3 inches below the navel and located closer to the navel than the spine. It is a point of focus for many meditative traditions.

[22] This point was stressed repeatedly during all of our conversations with Mr. Lo. He felt that a lifetime of dedication and practice are needed to master taijiquan, and effort and time devoted to other practices or martial arts merely take away resources needed to master taiji. After one has mastered taijiquan, then one may consider studying qigong or other martial arts.

Bibliography

Chen, W. (1929/1985). *T'ai chi ch'uan ta wen* [Questions and answers on t'ai chi ch'uan] (B. P. Lo & R. W. Smith, Trans.). Berkeley, CA: North Atlantic Books. (Original book published in Shanghai in 1929 and reprinted by the T'ai Chi Ch'uan Research Association of Taiwan, 1967).

Chen, X. (1919/1964). *Chen taijiquan tuishuo*. (Original book completed in 1919 and published by Chengshanmei Books, Taibei, Taiwan, 1984).

DeMarco, M. (1992). The origin and evolution of taijiquan. *Journal of Asian martial arts*, 1(1), 8–25.

Huang, W. (1979). *Fundamentals of t'ai chi ch'uan* (3rd. Ed.). Hong Kong: South Sky Book Company.

Jou, T. (1981). *The Tao of t'ai-chi ch'uan*. Warwick, NY: Tai Chi Foundation.

Liao, W. (1990). *T'ai chi classics*. Boston, MA: Shambhala.

Lo, B. (1985, August). Explanation of Tsuo-style tai chi chuan. *T'ai chi ch'uan*, issue no. 40, 8–14. (Published in Taiwan, translated into English by the author).

Lo, B., Inn, M., Amacker, R., & Foe, S. (1985). *The essence of t'ai chi ch'uan: The literary tradition*. Berkeley, CA: North Atlantic Books.

Lowenthal, W. (1994). *Gateway to the miraculous: Further explorations in the Tao of*

Cheng Man-ch'ing. Berkeley, CA: Frog, Ltd.

Seidel, A. (1970). A Taoist immortal of the Ming dynasty: Chang San-feng. In W. T. deBary (Ed.), *Self and society in Ming thought* (pp. 483–531). New York: Columbia University Press.

Smith, R. (1981a). *Pa-kua: Chinese boxing for fitness and self-defense*. New York: Kodansha International.

Smith, R. (1981b). *Hsing-i: Chinese mind-body boxing*. New York: Kodansha International.

Smith, R. (1995). Zheng Manqing and taijiquan: A clarification of role. *Journal of Asian martial arts, 4*(1), 50–65.

Smith, R. (1996). Han Qingtang and his seizing art. *Journal of Asian martial arts, 5*(1), 31–47.

Sun, T. (1988). *The art of war* (Thomas Cleary, Trans.). Boston: Shambhala.

Sutton, N. (1994). The development of Zheng Manqing taijiquan in Malaysia. *Journal of Asian martial arts, 3*(1), 56–71.

Wang, P., & Zeng, W. (1983). *Wu style taijiquan: A detailed course for health and self-defence and teachings of three famous masters in Beijing*. Hong Kong and Beijing: Hai Feng Publishing and Zhaohua Publishing.

Wu, D. (1984). *T'ai chi ch'uan yenchiu*. Hong Kong: Shangwu Books.

Wu, G. (1985). *T'ai chi ch'uan taochi*. Taibei: Shenlong Books.

Wu, J. (Ed.). (1979). *The pinyin Chinese-English dictionary*. Beijing: The Commercial Press.

Yang, J. (1982a). *Shaolin chin na: The seizing art of kung-fu*. Burbank, CA: Unique Publications.

Yang, J. (1982b). *Yang style tai chi chuan*. Burbank, CA: Unique Publications.

Yang, J. (1987). *Advanced Yang style tai chi chuan (vol. 1): Tai chi theory and tai chi jing*. Jamaica Plain, MA: Yang's Martial Arts Association.

Yang, J. (1989). *Muscle-tendon changing and marrow/brain washing chi kung: The secret of youth*. Jamaica Plain, MA: Yang's Martial Arts Association.

Yang, Z. (1988). *Yang style taijiquan*. Beijing and Hong Kong: Hai Feng Publishing and Morning Glory Press.

Zheng, M. (1950/1985). *Cheng Tzu's thirteen treatises on t'ai chi ch'uan* (B. P. Lo & M. Inn, Trans.). Berkeley, CA: North Atlantic Books. (Original book published in Taiwan in 1950).

Zheng, M. (1981). *Lao-Tzu: My words are very easy to understand*. Berkeley, CA: North Atlantic Books.

Zheng Manqing: The Memorial Hall and Legacy of the Master of Five Excellences in Taiwan

by Russ Mason, M.A.

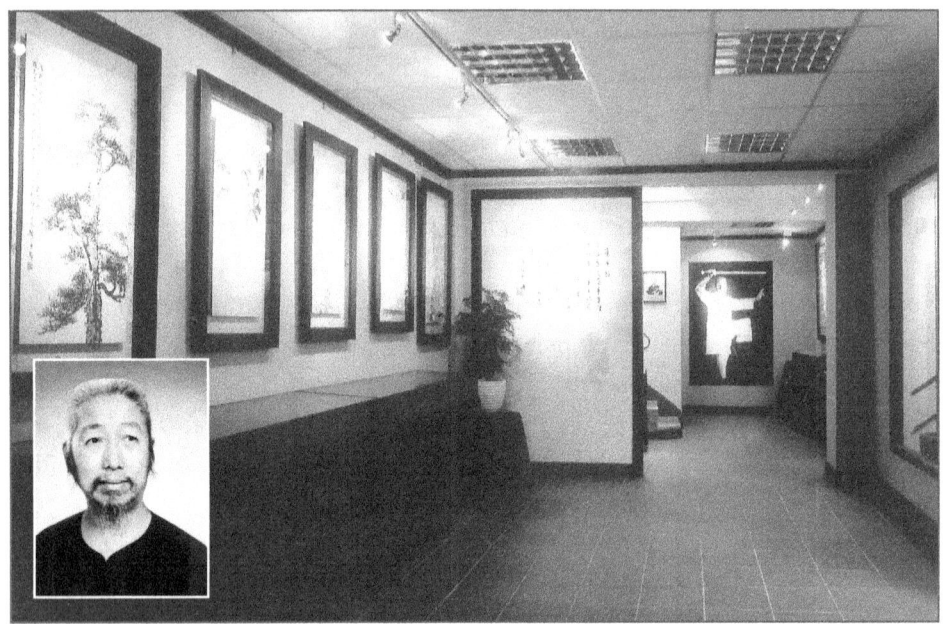

Inset photo of Professor Zheng courtesy of Robert W. Smith.
The large exhibit room in the downstairs area of the
Zheng Manqing Memorial Hall. It displays several
paintings and photographs of Professor Zheng.
Photo courtesy of Yuan Weiming.

Introduction

Professor Zheng Manqing (Cheng Man-ch'ing) has been called a "taiji genius" and a "multifaceted savant" (Smith, 1999: 201). A living bridge between ancient China and contemporary Western society, Zheng embodied the ideal of the cultivated Chinese gentleman of the literati class. In old China, a scholar needed a thorough knowledge of the literary classics, calligraphy, and poetry in order to pass the imperial civil service examinations, which were still in place during Zheng's childhood at the end of the Qing dynasty (1644–1911). These requirements of public office shaped the Chinese concept of education. Beyond these accomplishments a cultured man was expected to be familiar with painting, the game of Go (Weiqi), and other classical arts (Barnstone & Chou, 1996: xii). Zheng excelled in all of these arts. Moreover, following the Confucian ideal, Zheng blended the martial arts with the fine arts, for Confucius taught that without martial training (e.g., archery and charioteering) one could not master the mental discipline necessary for the civil arts (e.g., propriety, music, mathematics, and writing) (Zheng, 1985: 14).

Professor Zheng is known as the Master of Five Excellences, referring to his outstanding abilities in traditional Chinese medicine, martial arts, and fine arts (painting, poetry, and calligraphy). One American researcher has written that, in order to properly evaluate Zheng's accomplishments in the Chinese milieu, a westerner must begin by imagining a person who has made extraordinary contributions in classical scholarship, literary theory, and criticism. In addition, such a person is: "an Olympic boxer, president of a national medical association, distinguished poet and professor of literature, and [one whose] paintings hang in the Louvre" (Wile, 2007: 2). How did Professor Zheng establish a reputation of such stature that it is deserving of a memorial?

The following sections will present a concise biographical sketch of Zheng's early personal life, his academic and professional successes, and his training and accomplishments in the field of martial arts. The focus will be on his work in Taiwan, the growth of his Taibei school, and the posthumous establishment of the memorial hall currently housed in his former residence.

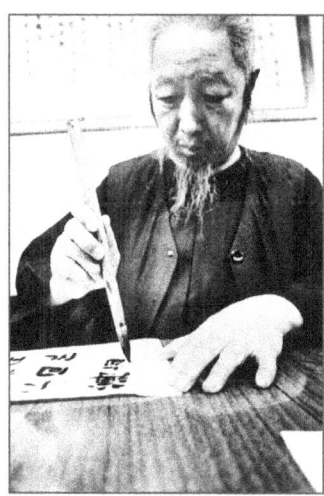

Professor Zheng completes a poem.
Photo courtesy of Ken van Sickle.

Early Life

Born in Yongjia County (now the Lucheng District of Wenzhou) in Zhejiang Province, Zheng Yue[1] grew up the youngest child in a family of humble means. His father died while he was still young, and life was hard. Yet, even as a child, Zheng's interest in calligraphy, painting, poetry, and medicinal herbs was encouraged and nurtured by his mother and maternal aunt. Yue was a precocious child with a keen and inquiring intellect who had memorized the Confucian classics by age nine. Then, after suffering a fracture of the skull in an accident, he spent two days and nights in a coma. A teacher of martial arts treated the boy with mountain herbs, and he regained consciousness but had completely lost his memory and was in a near vegetative state. His mother apprenticed Zheng soon after to local painter, Wang Xiangchan.[2] The simple, repetitive work of grinding ink proved therapeutic, and within five years the young artist had not only recovered his mental acuity, but had also mastered the skill of painting well enough to begin supporting himself and his family by selling his own works.

Academic and Professional Success

In 1916 the famed poet Lu Chengbei provided an introduction for the budding artist that led to further study in painting, poetry, and calligraphy in Hangzhou (Wile, 2007: 16). Three years later, at the tender age of seventeen, Zheng traveled to Beijing, where he met and was befriended by several elder painters and poets, winning their respect through his intelligence and skill. All around him young thinkers caught up in the May Fourth reform movement and the early days of the new republic were questioning the ancient ways, but Zheng's *guanxi* (social connections) with members of the older generation, developed through participation in these traditional artistic circles, led to an invitation to teach poetry at Yuwen University in Beijing (cir. 1919). Shortly afterward, Zheng received a recommendation to teach at National Jinan University in Shanghai from none other than Cai Yuanpei (1868–1940), one of the highest-ranking and most influential educators of the early Republican era (Davis, 1996: 40, 53). Cai was chancellor of Beijing University at that time. It is reasonable to assume that Cai's personal support opened doors and helped to propel the younger man's rapid rise in academia.

After his move south from the capital, Zheng became director of the painting department at the Shanghai School of Fine Arts and was also instrumental in establishing the College of Culture and Art there. But his responsibilities in Shanghai did not prevent him from mounting a solo art exhibition at Waterside (*Shuixie*) Pavilion in Beijing's Central Park, and in 1925, together with such colleagues as the famous artist Zhang Daqian, founding the Xiaohan Painting Society (Wile, 2007: 16). He also traveled to Japan to do research on the fine arts for the Chinese Ministry of Education (Davis, 1996: 40).

Zheng's students relate an anecdote[3] that clearly illustrates the young professor's artistic ability at this time in his career, as well as his photographic memory.

Once, while attending a dinner party at the home of the mayor of Shanghai, Zheng became fascinated by a hanging scroll created by a famous master of rattan painting. Stepping aside from the gathering of distinguished guests, he gazed long at the scroll, lost in admiration. When it was suggested that he might borrow the painting in order to study it in the privacy of his home, the young artist declined, saying that such extended study was unnecessary, as he had already committed the scene to memory. The next day Zheng presented a replica of the painting to his host. Mayor Wu was amazed to see that the replica painted by Zheng matched the original in every detail and was, in itself, a masterful work of art. After this, word of Zheng's artistic genius spread throughout Shanghai.

Some sources suggest Zheng's move to the south may have been partially motivated by health concerns, as he was already suffering from tuberculosis, which was aggravated by the northern Beijing climate as well as by the ubiquitous chalk dust of the classroom environment.[4] During his time in Shanghai, Zheng began to devote himself to a more serious study of Chinese medicine. Building on the foundational knowledge of herbal remedies gained from his mother, Zheng sought and gained tuition from Dr. Song You'an, a famous practitioner from Anhui Province who was persuaded to come out of retirement to provide a personal apprenticeship. Much later, Zheng practiced herbal medicine full time, eventually serving as president of the National Chinese Medical Association (Davis, 1996: 41). In addition to being named to the National Assembly for the Construction of the Constitution in 1946, Zheng was one year later elected to the National Assembly to represent the community of doctors of traditional Chinese medicine, a position he held until the end of his life (Cheng, 1971: 238).

Zheng Manqing was widely recognized as a man of great and varied accomplishments, so much so that Lin Sen (1868–1943), the Chairman of the Nationalist government at the time of the Sino-Japanese War, presented Zheng with a calligraphic inscription conferring upon him the title "Master of Five Arts."[5]

At the age of forty Zheng married Ding Yidu (known in the US as Madame Juliana T. Cheng), the daughter of General Ding Muhan, founder of the Chinese Air Force Bureau. Madame Zheng had been a student of medicine at Beijing University, and her specialty of medical practice became obstetrics. The couple would have five children.

Martial Accomplishments

Perhaps because of his childhood health concerns, Zheng early on studied exercises such as baduanjin and yijin (Davis, 1996: 40). He had also practiced taijiquan intermittently beginning in 1923 in an attempt to bolster his weak physique, but each time his physical condition would improve, he would leave off practice to devote himself to other endeavors.⁶ After Zheng's tuberculosis progressed to the point of coughing up blood, he committed himself to persevere in a daily exercise regimen. Zheng received an introduction to the famous master Yang Chengfu and credited the practice of Yang-style taijiquan with his complete recovery from the life-threatening illness (Cheng, 1971: 238, Cheng, 1985: 64; and Yang, 1934/2005: 2).

In his own book, Yang Zhenji (Yang Chengfu's second son; b. 1921) emphasized the fact that Zheng was his father's disciple and that Zheng was the scholar who transcribed Yang Chengfu's 1934 book, *The Essence and Applications of Taijiquan* (*Taijiquan tiyong quanshu*) (Yang, 1993: 250). In addition to being chosen to record Yang's teaching, Zheng was further honored by being asked to write a preface for the master's book.⁷

One of Yang Chengfu's senior-most students was Li Yaxuan. Li's student, Yan Changkong, writes that after the Maoist victory, subsequent editions of Yang's book censored Zheng's name and preface for political reasons. This was due to his connections with Chiang Kai-shek. However, after thirty years of blackout, Zheng's name and biography are once again appearing in mainland publications (Wile, 2007: 15, 32; Davis, 1996: 48). Yan also recorded Li's statement that Yang gave Zheng private instruction in inner cultivation (neigong), which helped him comprehend the subtler elements of the art. Yan, citing Li Yaxuan's high standards, went on to note that Li's praise for Zheng's insights and skills was "truly a rare thing" (Wile, 2007: 33, 35).

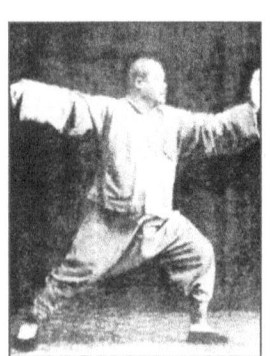 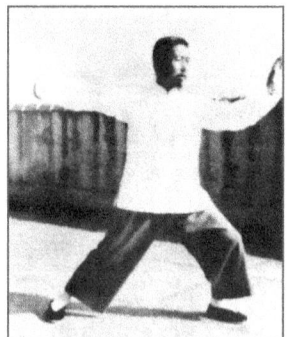 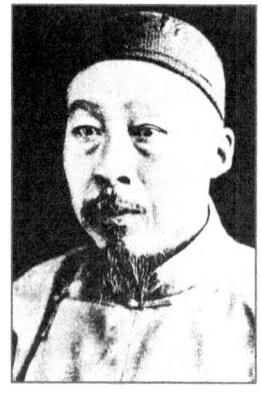

Left to right: Yang Chengfu (ca. 1933)
and his student Zheng Manqing (ca. 1948)
show the posture of single whip. Chen Weiming,
a senior student of Yang Chengfu and a classmate,
friend, and supporter of Zheng Manqing.

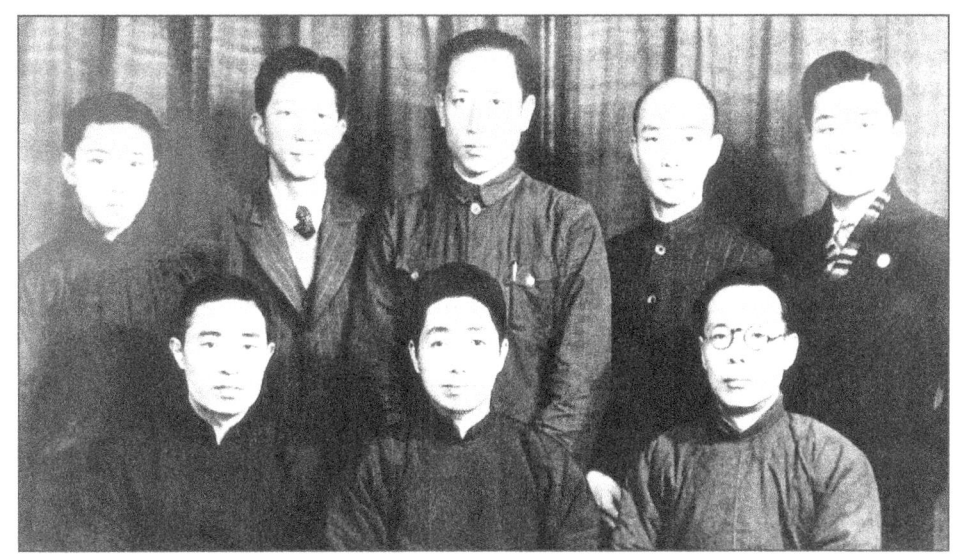

Professor Zheng Manqing (center front) in China in 1943
with a group of students: directly behind Zheng is
Zhang Zigang; in the rear row, far right with scarf,
is Guo Qingfang, Western boxing lightweight
champion of China in the late 1930s.
Photo courtesy of Guo Qingfang.

Another of Yang's most famous students was Chen Weiming (1881–1958). Chen was not only a senior student of Yang Chengfu, but also a scholar and writer who had himself represented Yang's teachings in print.[8] After the Sino-Japanese war, Zheng took the early manuscript of his own text, *Master Zheng's Thirteen Treatises on Taijiquan*, to Chen to see whether it would meet with his senior classmate's approval (Cheng, 1965/1999: 9). Zheng felt that both his book and his approach to taijiquan were merely a continuation of Yang's own teaching and earlier text, *Essence and Applications of Taijiquan*. Chen approved of Zheng's work and urged its publication, even offering to write a preface (Cheng, 1985: 108; Cheng, 1965/1999: 9). Chen wrote in his preface to the book that, during the years of Zheng's study, when Madame Yang (née Hou) fell ill, Zheng used his knowledge of herbal medicine to treat her, saving her life. Chen writes: "Master Yang was so thankful that he taught [Zheng] all the secret oral transmissions. No one else had ever heard them" (Wile, 1985: 1). Chen supported Zheng's conviction that an overarching principle of Yang-style taijiquan is commitment to the twin principle: sink-relax (*chen song*), something that would come to be a distinguishing characteristic of Zheng's approach to taijiquan.[9]

Fu Zhongwen (1903–1994, nephew, disciple, and teaching assistant of Yang Chengfu) stated that Zheng established his reputation in the 1930s in Yang's circle because of his deep interest in tuishou (pushing hands) and his enthusiastic training with the most skilled seniors (Yu & Sharp, 1993: 45–46). After developing his skill by working with Yang and his senior students, Zheng went on to meet a number of public and private challenges, some involving British and American military personnel and others with well-regarded Chinese boxers. The fact that Zheng served as head of the Hunan Martial Arts Academy (as well as serving on the faculty of two other military academies) and the fact that he won the respect of the seasoned military officers he worked with attest to the functionality of his skills.[10]

On the mainland, Zheng was called upon in 1933 to teach taijiquan to Nationalist troops at the Central Military Academy (formerly known as Huangpu). Later, during the Sino-Japanese War, he taught in Sichuan for the Central Military Training Group (Davis, 1996: 41). In 1938, as director of the provincial government's Hunan Martial Arts Academy, Zheng was responsible for training hundreds of officers in only two months' time. Under these circumstances he was forced to simplify the Yang-style long form by eliminating repetitions, eventually settling on thirty-seven as the standard number of postures for his version of the solo exercise.[11]

Arrival in Taiwan

After the surrender of Japan in 1945, full-scale civil war reerupted in China between the Nationalist forces of Generalissimo Chiang Kai-shek (the Guomindang) and the Maoists. After the communist victory on the mainland in 1949, Zheng immigrated to Taiwan with the Guomindang. Eventually, he settled in a house on Zhongxing Road in Yunghe, a suburb of Chiang Kai-shek's capital city, Taibei. He would dub the place Xi Chang Lou, which could be interpreted "Tower of Long Evening" or "Long Night Lodge" (Wile, 2007: 52). There he concentrated on practicing medicine, later opening a taijiquan school on the top floor of Zhongshan Hall at the request of Taibei mayor You Mijian (Wile, 2007: 18). In Taiwan, Zheng taught his thirty-seven-posture simplified form (*jianyi taijiquan*) publicly to civilians.

After establishing himself as a physician in Taiwan, Zheng accepted his first student on the island in the art of taijiquan. Benjamin Lo, a young university student, came for medical treatment and was advised to practice taijiquan so his body could develop the strength needed to absorb the prescribed herbal medications (Davis & Mann, 1996: 50).[12] Beginning in 1949, Lo went to Professor Zheng's home each day to learn taijiquan in the traditional way, perfecting the form posture by posture. He would later come to the United States, where he has taught Zheng's method since 1974. Soon after Lo began to study, Liu Xiheng bowed as a disciple to Zheng, followed by Xu Yizhong and others. As the master's fame spread throughout the island, many more students were added, most coming with previous training in the martial arts and, in the traditional way, by personal introduction. Zheng established the Shizhong Study Society (Shizhong Xueshe)[13] in 1949 for the promotion of taijiquan (Davis, 1996: 43; Wile, 2007: 7; see also the Shizhong webpage).

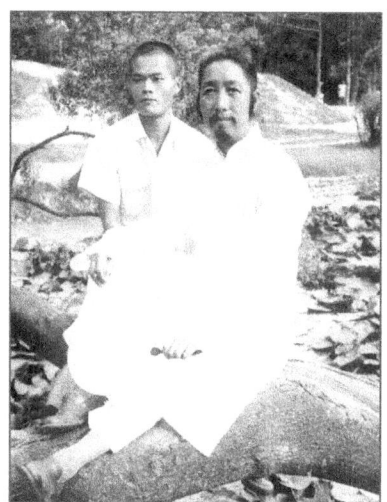 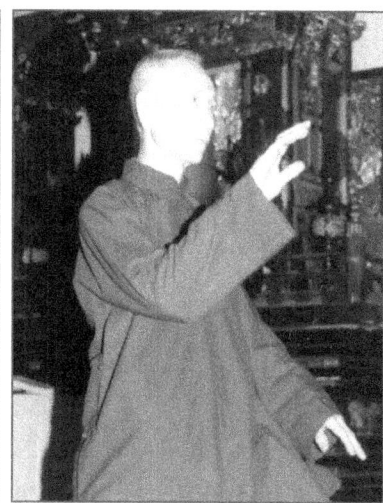

Zheng Manqing with his first student in Taiwan,
Benjamin Lo, in the botanical garden, Taibei, 1951.
Photo courtesy of Benjamin Lo.
Liu Xiheng shows brush knee twist step.
Photo courtesy of Liu Xiheng.

In addition to heading his own school, the Shizhong Study Society, Zheng was a member of the Chinese Taijiquan Club (Zhong Guo Taijiquan Ju Le Bu), formally established on March 27, 1960. National assembly member Chen Panling (who was also head of the ROC Chinese Boxing Association) served as chief commissioner. In addition to Zheng and Chen, other well-known members included Wang Yannian, Xiong Yanghe, Guo Lianyin, and Han Qingtang. Later, in 1963, an expanded version of the club, known as the Taijiquan Academic Research Committee, was established under the auspices of the Sino-American Cultural and Economic Association, with Zheng serving as a consultant (Fairchild & Lin, 2007: 2–3).

During the period between 1959 and 1962, American martial arts historian Robert W. Smith was assigned a CIA post in Taiwan as intelligence advisor to the admiral of the US Pacific Fleet. His research into the practice and history of Chinese martial arts led him to Zheng's door and, eventually, to a lifelong commitment to Zheng's taijiquan method.[14] As Zheng's first Western student, Smith did much to publicize "the Professor" (as he was respectfully addressed by his students) in the West. In 1964 Zheng traveled abroad, first to Paris and then to the United States, where he exhibited his paintings at the Cernuschi Museum of Chinese Art and the Republic of China pavilion of the New York World's Fair, respectively.[15] After establishing a residence in New York City, Zheng received the title director of fine arts, the Republic of China Cultural Renaissance Movement, American Branch from the Chiang Kai-shek government (Davis, 1996: 46). There he established an American branch of his Shizhong School to promote taijiquan, as well as other forms of traditional Chinese arts and culture. Leaving Liu Xiheng in charge of his school in Taiwan in his absence (Davis, 1996: 54), Zheng would balance his time between his homes in New York and Taibei over the next ten years. During this period he exhibited paintings at the FAR Gallery in 1968 and at the Hudson River Museum in 1973 and authored some of his most profound works, including commentaries on the *Daodejing*, the *Yijing*, and the Confucian classics of the *Analects*, the *Great Learning*, and the *Doctrine of the Mean* (Cheng, 1971/1981: 239; Davis, 1996: 46). At this time in his life, Zheng led flourishing taijiquan schools in both America and the Republic of China. His work did much to popularize taijiquan in the West and Taiwan, and to establish the international reputation of his thirty-seven-posture simplified Yang-style short form. Professor Zheng was particularly noted in the international martial arts community for his remarkable skill in push-hands (tuishou).

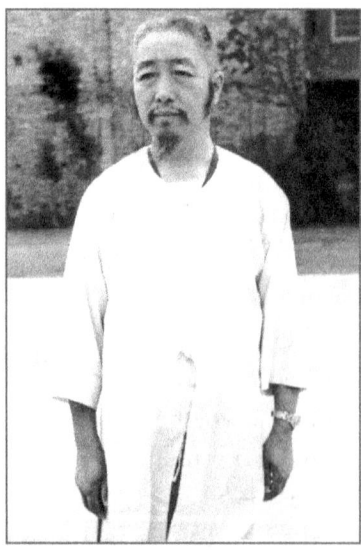

Zheng Manqing (1902–1975).

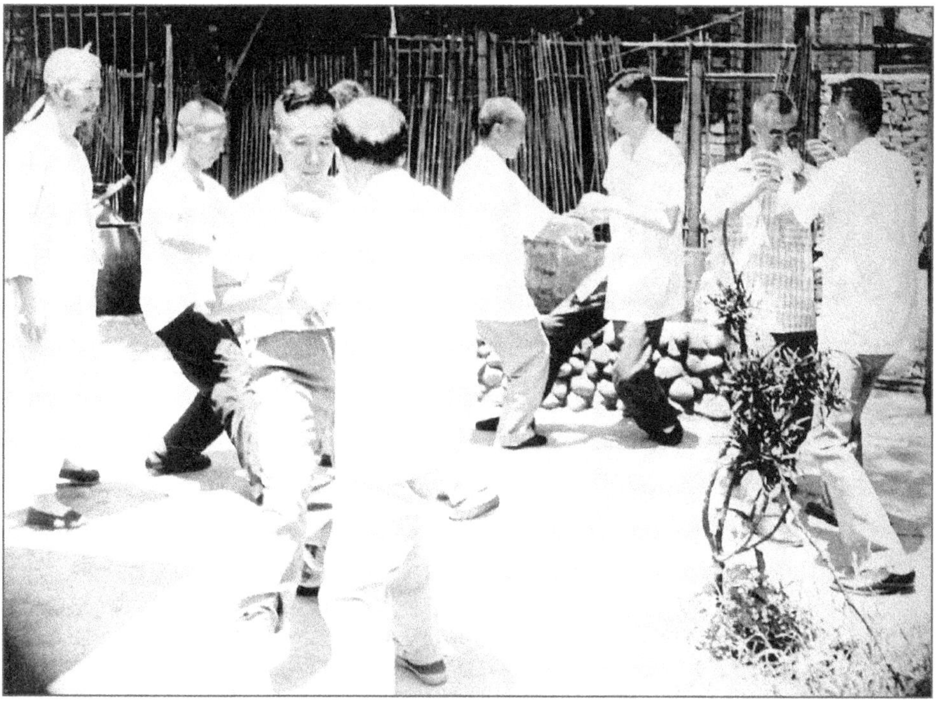

Professor Zheng watches students
push hands at his residence in Yonghe.

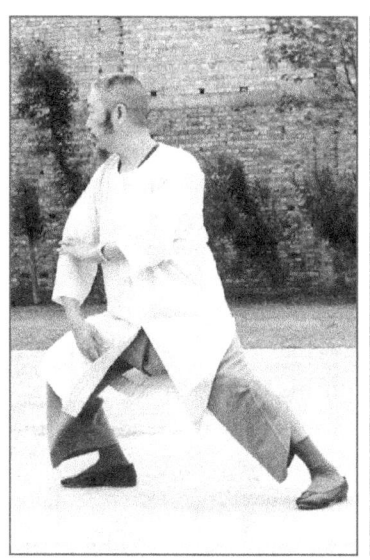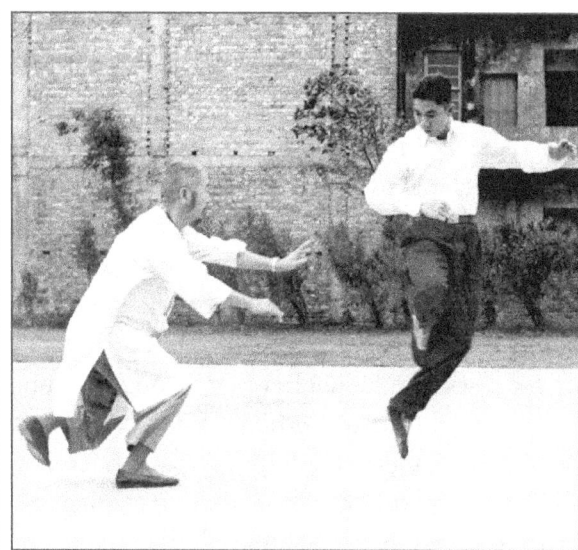

In the posture shoulder stroke. Repelling an attacker. Note the
cross-substantial push: rooted right foot and active left hand.

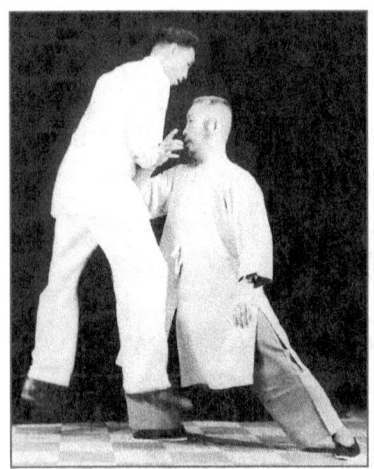 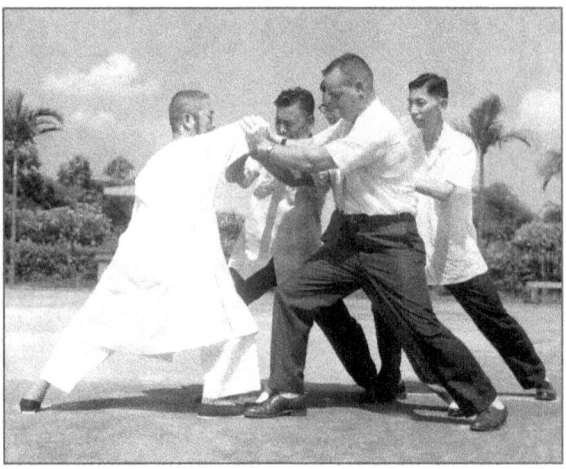

Left: Zheng Manqing uproots William C. C. Chen.
Note the relaxed hands and the effective *tifang* (lit: lift/let-go).
Withstands the push of four men (Taiwan, c. 1960).
Photos courtesy of Robert W. Smith.

Zheng's Death and Legacy in Taiwan

Zheng died on March 26, 1975, from the effects of a cerebral hemorrhage suffered at his home in Taibei (Wile, 2007: 19). The Master of the Five Excellences funeral was attended by hundreds, including distinguished representatives from his many fields of endeavor, students, and government officials. Memorials were also held in Singapore and New York City (Davis 1996: 48).

Upon Professor Zheng's passing, Liu Xihong succeeded him as president of the Taibei Shizhong Study Society in 1975 and served in this capacity, heading up taijiquan instruction at the school, until his retirement in 1986. His classmate, Xu Yizhong, served as president after that. In addition, in 1993 Xu was elected first committee chairman of a new organization, the Master Zheng Taijiquan Study Association. Chairman Xu served the first two consecutive terms at this post. Ke Qihua served as third committee chairman from 1999 until his passing in 2001, with Ju Hongbin of Gaoxiong finishing out his term.[16] Following this, Xu Yizhong returned to the post and continues to serve in this capacity at the present time. Current advisors to the association include two names familiar to the American taijiquan community: Benjamin P. Lo and William C. C. Chen. With the assistance of his able advisors and instructors, the association chairman, Xu Yizhong, is tireless in his efforts to promote Professor Zheng's simplified taijiquan in Taiwan and around the world.

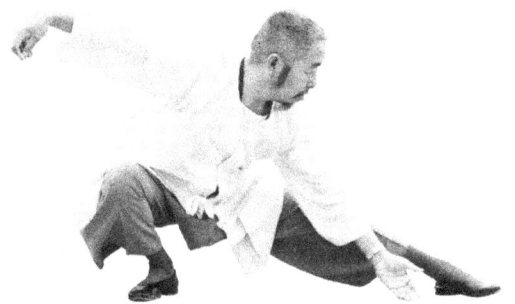
Zheng shows the posture squatting single whip.

Among the special events organized by the association was the hundredth anniversary celebration of Professor Zheng Manqing's birth. This week-long event was celebrated in August of 2000 and featured panel discussions, martial arts demonstrations, a tournament, and an exhibition of Zheng's paintings and calligraphy on loan from the National Palace Museum.[17]

Today simplified taijiquan has come full circle, as one of Zheng's senior students in Taiwan, Chairman Xu Yizhong, traveled in October of 2006 to Nankai University in Tianjin on the Chinese mainland to teach the form at the request of that university's martial arts (wushu) community. Nankai University's curriculum currently offers an ongoing course to research Professor Zheng's simplified taijiquan, and other such programs are in the discussion stage. In addition, the Beijing University of Physical Education and related organizations have expressed interest in publishing Zheng's instructional books on taijiquan.[18]

Establishment of the Zheng Manqing Memorial Hall

In the years following Professor Zheng's passing, Madame Juliana T. Zheng and her family continued to divide their time between the United States and Taiwan, using the old home place on Zhongxing Road in Yonghe as a base during their visits to Taibei. After Madame Zheng's passing in January 2005, it was decided that a portion of the family residence would be refurbished and converted to a memorial hall for the preservation of Professor Zheng's artifacts and legacy. After much work on the part of the family, students, Chairman Xu Yizhong, and the association, the opening ceremony of the Zheng Manqing Memorial Hall was celebrated on June 25, 2006. Due to space limitations and the number of guests, the ceremony was held in the gymnasium of the Taibei Wuchang Junior High School (the current location of taijiquan classes offered by the Shizhong Study Society). In attendance were five hundred people, including noted artists, poets, philosophers, and the head of the Taiwan National Taijiquan Association, Zhan Deshen.

Xu Chongming (the first chair advisor of the Zhengzi Taijiquan Study Association) made a report of Master Zheng's history in Taiwan, and Chou Bozi (the vice chairman of the committee) presented a golden key to the new memorial hall facility.[19] In November of 2006, this author visited the memorial hall. The photographic tour of the Zheng Manqing Memorial Hall outlined here is presented with the permission of Chairman Xu and the assistance of the association staff and others. Visitors to the memorial are welcome and may receive further information by visiting www.37taichi.org.tw. In addition, plans are under consideration to offer overseas memberships in the association. For more information on becoming a member to the memorial, please contact the association at www.37taichi@yahoo.com.tw.

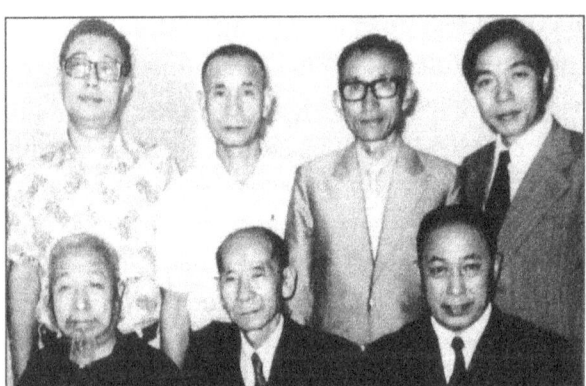 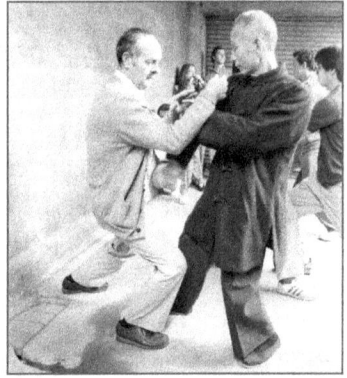

Above, left: Zheng with friends and senior students. First row, left to right: Zheng, Mr. Hong (friend and legal advisor from Hong Kong), and Wang Yannian. Back row, left to right: Mr. Yang (a lawyer friend), Liu Xiheng (first president of the association), the late Tao Bingxiang (d. 2006), and Xu Yizhong (current president of the association). Right: Liu Xiheng and Robert W. Smith push hands in Taibei (1983). Photo courtesy of Robert W. Smith.

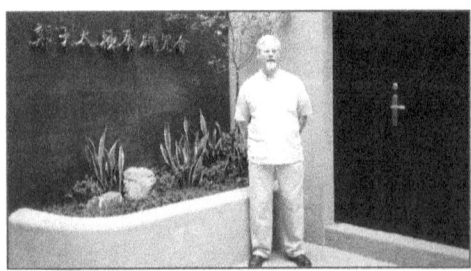 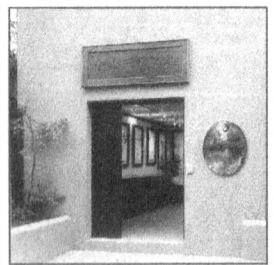

Danny Emerick stands outside the door to the memorial hall at the Professor's old residence. The entranceway with sign above reading Zheng Manqing Memorial Hall. Photos by R. Mason.

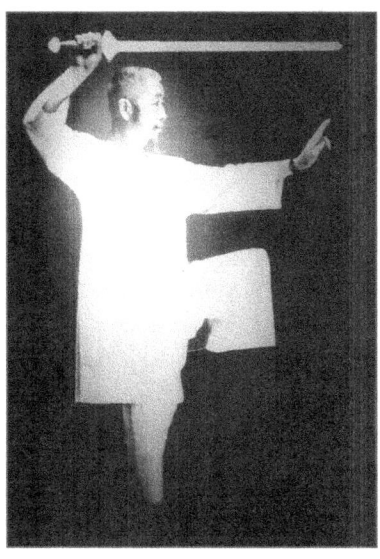 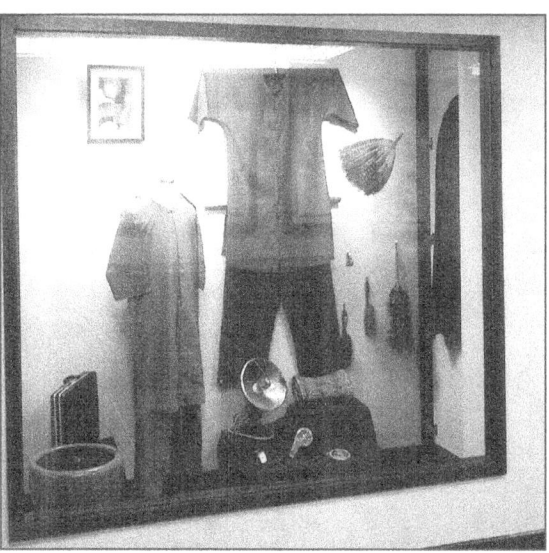

Above left: Zheng with sword in the posture of major literary star (*da kui xing*). Photo by R. Mason. Right: A display case containing Zheng's personal artifacts. Next to this is also a brief lineage chart, and a chronology of his life. Photo courtesy of Yuan Weiming.

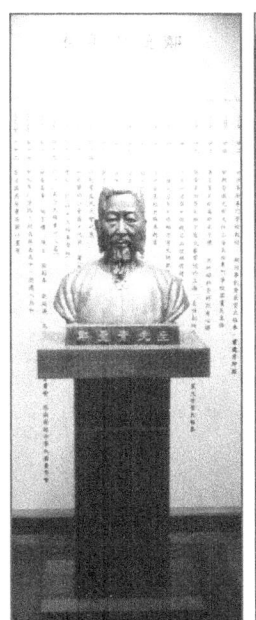 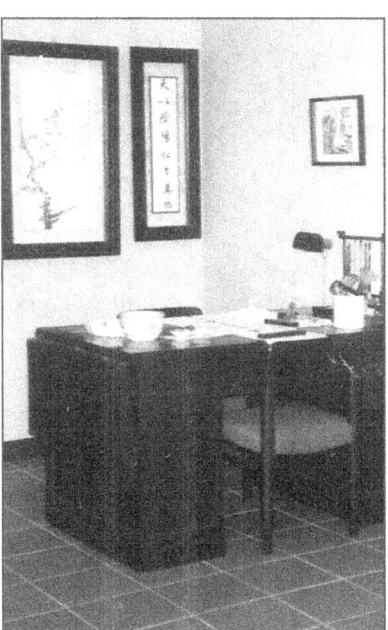 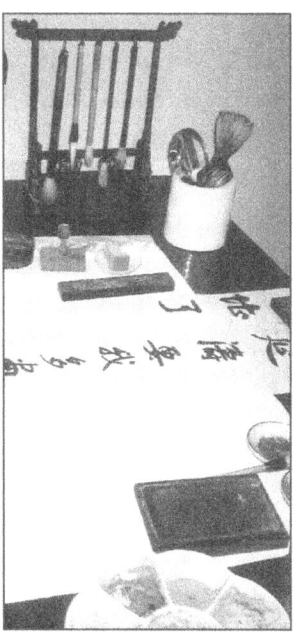

Above left: This life-size bronze bust of Professor Zheng stands in a small alcove with a chronology of his major life events. Center and right: Zheng's desk and details of the desktop showing inkstone, brushes, calligraphy, and personal name seal (chop). Photos by R. Mason.

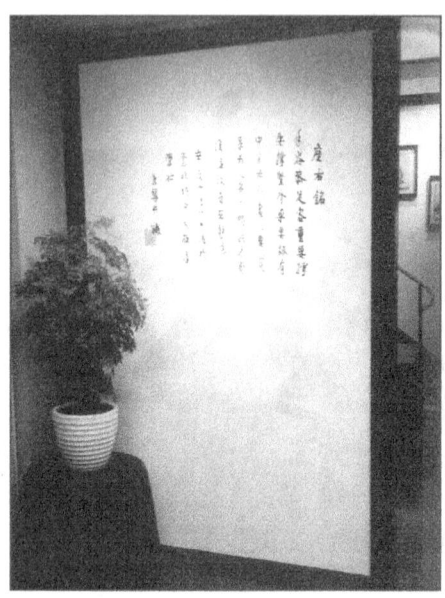

Zheng's *zuo you ming* calligraphy
superimposed over a photo of him in the
posture single whip. Photos by R. Mason.

Zheng Manqing's Zuo You Ming

As one enters the front door of the memorial hall, straight ahead and toward the left wall is a large panel displaying a 1949 photograph of Zheng in the single-whip posture. Overlaid on the photo is his *zuo you ming* calligraphy. The terms *zuo you* literally translate "seat right hand," and *ming* can be interpreted "inscription," "tablet," or "motto." Therefore, the phrase "zuo you ming" could refer to something that is carved and kept close at hand for constant reference, as in "words to live by." Written in the terse, classical style, the verses of Zheng's poem resonate with literary allusion and could be interpreted in various ways. The gist of the motto goes something like this:

> Allow the hands to be led lightly and humbly;
> Allow the feet to be heavy, stepping with dignity.
> Hang straight; hang straight! Be poised and upright.
> Speak sparingly, directly, and with great care;
> Be forgiving and generous; out of a centered heart, give back.
> Be loyal, tolerant, and patient in your dealings;
> Let your attitude toward others be temperate.
> Repent, and correct your errors with silent contemplation.

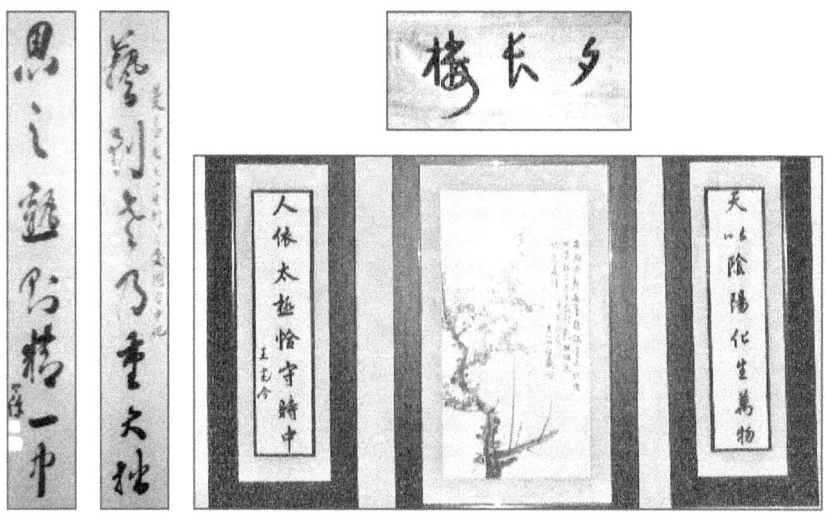

Left to right: Red scrolls constituting a matching couplet. Blossoming bough flanked by a matching couplet. Above these is a wooden plaque with Zheng's Tower of Long Evening calligraphy. All photos by R. Mason.

Matching Couplet Red Scrolls

Upstairs, on either side of the entryway between the conference room and Professor Zheng's office, hang two red vertical scrolls of verse. The pair constitutes a poem of a special structure called *duilian*. In such paired scrolls, the Chinese phrasing and grammar must match exactly; therefore, the creation of this type of verse is very demanding. The two sections of the couplet depicted here read something like this:

> When you ponder deeply, you will reach high
> competency in the area of your special skill.
> When your artistic skill has reached maturity,
> You will plumb the depths of great simplicity.

Matching Couplet with Blossoming Bough

Behind Professor Zheng's desk hangs a painting of a blossoming bough. Above the painting is a wooden plaque with the inscription "Tower of Long Evening" (Xi Chang Lou), Zheng's nickname for his study. On either side of the painting is another couplet. The couplet reads:

> Heaven creates all living things from yin and yang.
> All humanity depends upon taiji to safeguard Shizhong.

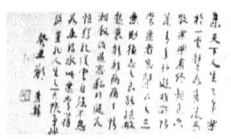 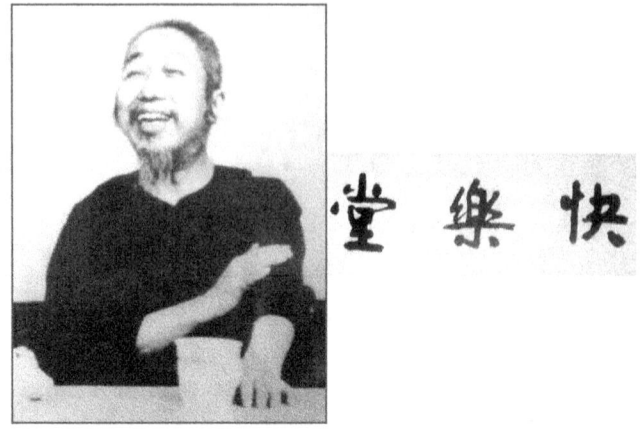

"Hall of Happiness" calligraphy. Professor Zheng expounds with a smile. Photo by R. Mason.

The Hall of Happiness
On this broad, horizontal work of calligraphy, Professor Zheng's beautiful brushwork showcases his poem "The Hall of Happiness" (*"Tang Le Kuai"*). The text of the poem appears below as translated by Tam Gibbs:

> May the joy that is everlasting gather in this hall. Not the joy of a sumptuous feast, which slips away even as we leave the table; nor that which music brings—it is only of a limited duration. Beauty and a pretty face are like flowers; they bloom for a while, then die. Even our youth slips swiftly away and is gone. No; enduring happiness is not in these, nor in the three joys of Tung Kung. We may as well forget them, for the joy I mean is worlds away from these. It is the joy of continuous growth, of helping to develop in ourselves and others the talents and abilities with which we were born—the gifts of heaven to mortal men. It is to revive the exhausted and to rejuvenate that which is in decline so that we are enabled to dispel sickness and suffering. Let true affection and happy concourse abide in this hall. Let us here correct our past mistakes and lose preoccupation with self. With the constancy of the planets in their courses or of the dragon in his cloud-wrapped path, let us enter the land of health and ever after walk within its bounds. Let us fortify ourselves against weakness and learn to be self-reliant, without ever a moment's lapse. Then our resolution will become the very air we breathe, the world we live in; then we will be as happy as a fish in crystal waters. This is the joy which lasts, that we can carry with us to the end of our days. And tell me, if you can; what greater happiness can life bestow?

Ying Erpo's Stylized Calligraphy of Zheng Kung

Hanging in the larger ground-floor room to the left of the display case is a specialized piece of artwork created by Ying Erpo. It consists of a stylized character for the family name Zheng in the form of a painting of Professor Zheng preparing to perform the posture turn body and sweep lotus with leg. The figure is like a riddle, with various parts of the body made up of stylized strokes from the character. The inscription to the right of the image reads:

> Taijiquan's founder Zhang Sanfeng's
> true successor Master Zheng Manqing's
> 'name-character' is here stylized into
> this figure in memory of the inauguration
> of the Master Zheng Manqing Memorial
> Hall on this 25th day of June (Zheng's
> birthday) in the year 2006.

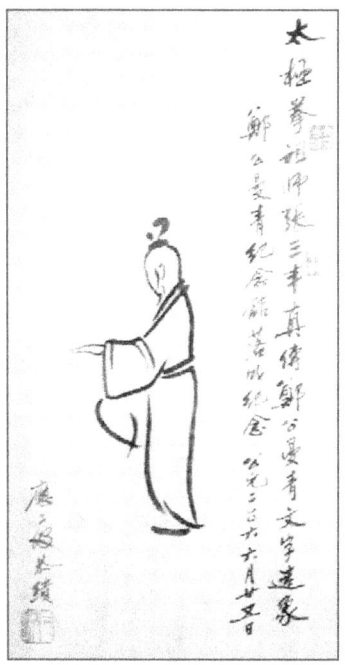

Ying Erpo's stylized painting
of the character *zheng* (鄭).
Photo by R. Mason.

The inscription to the bottom left reads: "Respectfully drawn by Ying Erpo."

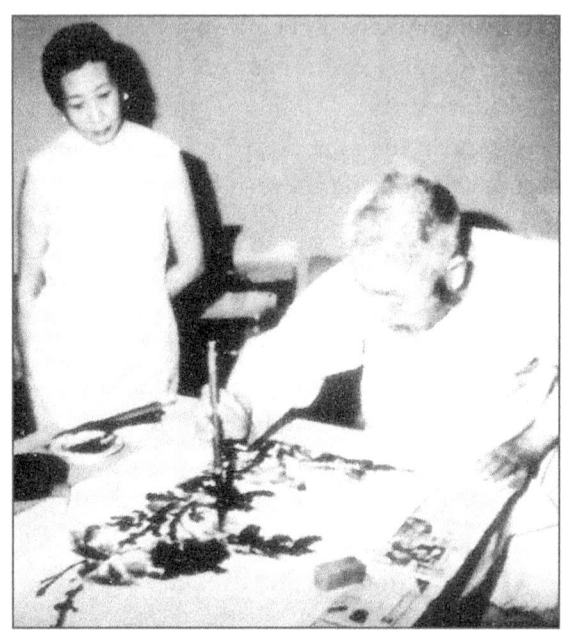

Professor Zheng does brushwork as Madame Zheng looks on.
Courtesy of the Zheng Manqing Memorial Hall.

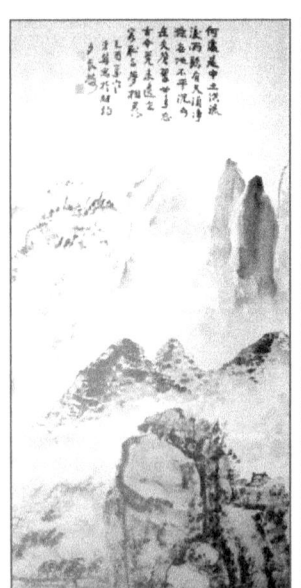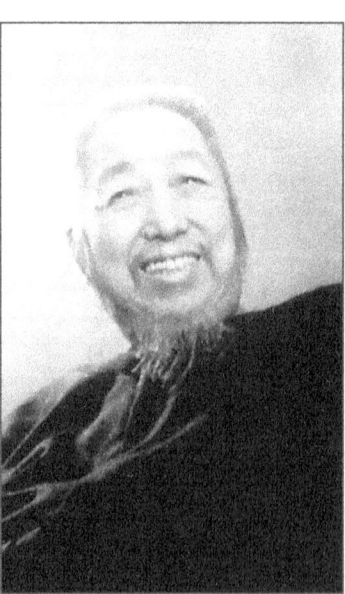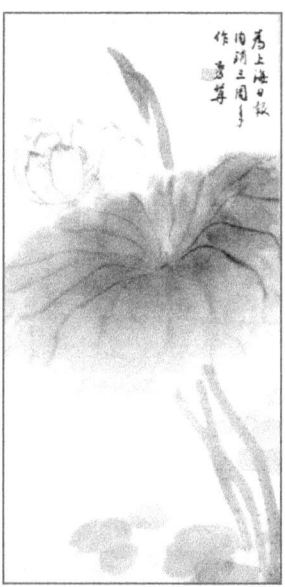

Examples of Professor Zheng's paintings:
a mountain landscape (left) and a single
lotus (right). Center: Zheng relaxing.

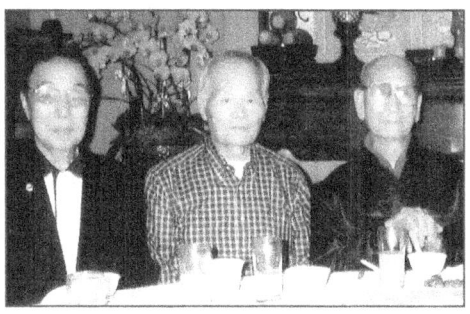 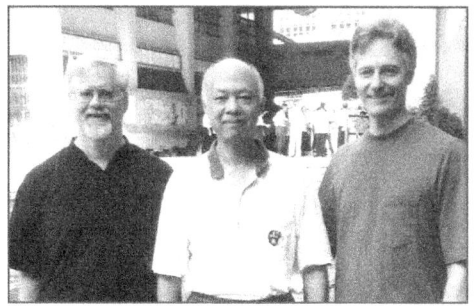

Left: Three of Professor Zheng's most senior students, left to right: current president Xu Yizhong, association advisor Benjamin Lo, and first president Liu Xiheng. Photo courtesy of Danny Emerick.
Right: Shizhong instructor Yuan Weiming with Danny Emerick and the author. Taijiquan classes at Wu Chang Junior High School facility are in progress in the background.

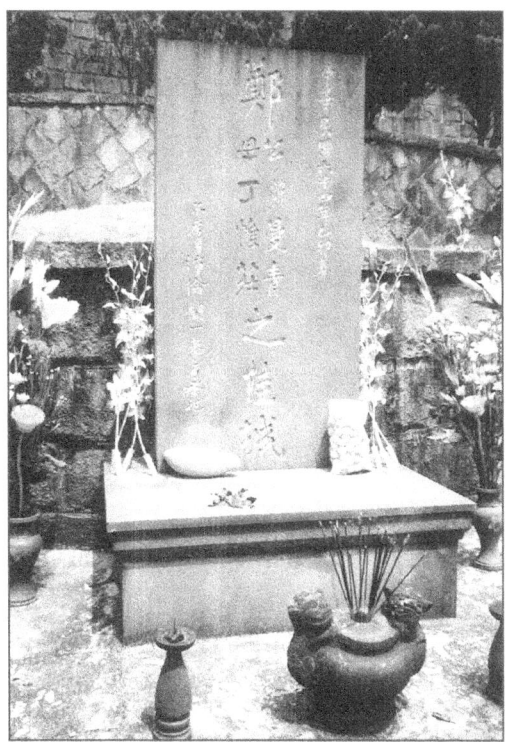

Professor Zheng Manqing's tombstone, Taibei, Taiwan.
Photo courtesy of Mark Westcott.

Glossary			
Chen Zhicheng (William C. C.)	陳至誠	Shi Zhong Xueshe	时中學社
Chen Panling	陳泮嶺	Tang Le Kuai	堂樂快
Chen Weiming	陳微明	Tao Bingxiang	陶炳祥
duilian	對聯	tuishou	推手
Fu Zhongwen	傅鍾文	Xiong Yanghe	熊養和
guanxi	關係	Xu Yizhung	徐憶中
Li Yaxuan	李雅軒	Yang Chengfu	楊澄甫
Liang Tongcai	梁棟材	Yang Jianho	楊健侯
Lin Sen	林森	Yang Shaohou	楊少侯
Liu Xiheng	劉錫亨	Yonghe City	永和市
Luo Bangzhen (Benjamin Lo)	羅邦楨	Zheng Manqing	鄭曼青
neigong	內功	Zheng Yue	鄭岳
Zheng Manqing Jinian Guan		鄭曼青 紀念 館	

Notes

1. Although Yue was his given name, later in life Zheng would adopt the sobriquet Manqing. Other nicknames and titles would be conferred upon him by others, and he would adopt a variety of pen names. See Yan Changkong's "Recollections of Zheng" (Wile, 2007: 32), Min Xiaoji's comments in his brief biography of "Man-Jan" (Cheng, 1985: 13–15), and Barbara Davis (1996: 39) for more biographical details.
2. Professor Zheng's American assistant and translator, Tam Gibbs, provides details in the brief biography of Zheng appended to his translation of Zheng's commentary on Laozi (Cheng, 1971: 237). Barbara Davis cites the *Great Dictionary of Names and Aliases of Contemporary and Modern China* as a source of details on Wang Xiangchan, whose given name was Ruyuan and who was known for his flower and plant paintings, the specialization that would become Zheng's forte (Davis, 1996: 39, 53).
3. This story was related to the author by Benjamin Lo in a conversation on April 29, 2007. A version of the story also appears in an article by Xu Yizhong, translated into English by Douglas Wile (2007: 29).
4. See Liang Tongcai's remarks recorded by Robert W. Smith (1974: 29) and Professor Zheng's own writings on his recovery from lung disease (Cheng, 1985: 64).
5. See Yan Changkong's remarks (Wile, 2007: 32).
6. Zheng discusses his early, sporadic practice and his ultimate commitment and perseverance in his book (Cheng, 1962: 25), as well as in his preface to Yang

Chengfu's *Essence and Applications of Taijiquan* (Yang, 1934/2005, 1–2).

7   The fact that Zheng worked with Yang Chengfu, transcribing the master's words for his final literary opus, has been acknowledged by Yang's sons, as well as other independent sources. Gu Liuxin, the president of the Shanghai Martial Arts Association, states the fact of Zheng's contribution in his introduction to Yang Zhenduo's book on Yang-style taijiquan (Yang, 1988: 8). Prefaces written by Yang Shouzhong and Zheng Manqing, as well as a discussion of Zheng's contributions to the wording and presentation of Yang Chengfu's teaching, may be read in Louis Swaim's 2005 English translation of Yang's masterwork (Yang, 1934/2005). See also (Mason, 2006) for a review of Swaim's translation. The Taiwan edition of Yang Zhengguo's book, *Yang Style Tai Chi Clearly Explained*, contains a preface by Zheng's student Xu Yizhong.

8   See Chen's 1929 work, translated into English in 1985 by Benjamin Lo and Robert W. Smith, in which Chen presents the teaching of his master, Yang Chengfu (Chen, 1929/1985: 11–12).

9   Like Chen Weiming, Zheng insisted that in real taijiquan one must not use even the slightest force; one must have utter faith in the principle of relaxing body and mind totally (Cheng & Smith, 1967: 101). Following Yang Chengfu, Chen Weiming also wrote that those who insist on using force never obtain the essence of taijiquan: "They can't believe that at the limit of suppleness lies a different quality of strength" (Chen, 1929/1985: 18). Yang Chengfu told Zheng continuously that he must relax completely, not using the slightest force to defend himself. Only by "investing in loss" in this way can one manifest Laozi's maxim that "The soft and pliable will defeat the hard and strong" (Cheng, 1985: 22, 87–88). Yang Chengfu's emphasis on softness reiterates the teaching of his own father, Yang Jianhou: "The first step in learning taijiquan martial applications is learning how to be light and agile. That means without muscular force" (Yang, 2001: 3), which in turn echoes the words of the *Taiji Classics*: "The softest will become the strongest" (Lo/Inn/Amacker/Foe, 1979: 19, 32, 37, 46, etc.).

10 In an interview (Mason, 2001) Robert W. Smith noted that, in his personal experience with taijiquan exponents, there was no one equal to Zheng. Smith hastened to add, however, that in saying this he was not maintaining that Zheng was the best in China. By Zheng's own admission, others even in the Yang Chengfu circle such as Li Yaxuan and Zhang Qinlin were superior to him in tuishou (Mason, 2001, Vol. 10, No. 1: 42). For accounts of Zheng's challenge matches, see Zheng's writings, as well as articles and books by others, particularly Liang Tongcai, Robert W. Smith, and Douglas Wile. Liang Tongcai claimed to have studied with fifteen different teachers of taijiquan, including direct students of Yang Chienhou, Yang Banhou, and Yang Shaohou, yet, like Smith, Liang maintained that Zheng was the greatest master of taijiquan he had ever personally encountered. Other evidence supports

the legitimacy of Zheng's skills (see Hayward, 1993: 94; Wile, 2007: 24–25; Smith, 1974/1990: 37–42, Smith, 1999: 196–197, 304; Smith, 1995, Vol. 4, No. 3, etc.).

11 Zheng discusses his reasons for abbreviating the Yang family form in his essay entitled "Taijiquan and Physical Education" in the section "In Martial Arts Seek Quality Not Quantity" (Wile, 2007: 103–104, see also p. 80) and also in his 1965 work (Cheng, 1965/1999: 9). Zheng's use of the number thirty-seven is noteworthy and not without precedent. Chen Weiming, in his 1929 text, selected photos of a number of important postures for practice, citing as precedent that "Long ago [Xu Xianbing] taught an exercise of thirty-seven-postures, discrete and unconnected" (Chen, 1929/1985: 12). Yang Banhou refers to the thirty-seven postures of Yang-style taijiquan in his song "Nine Key Secrets of Taijiquan" (Yang, 2001: 7). [Xu Longhou] offers one theory of taiji's origin in which there was a hermit named [Xu Xuanbing] who lived in Anhuei Province during the Tang dynasty and created a style of taijiquan named Thirty-Seven, after the movements of his form (see Smith, 1974/1990: 115; and Jou, 1981/1991: 8–9). Although Zheng does not explain the significance of the number, one may assume it is noteworthy, as varied listings of postures appear in the books authored by Zheng, yet the total number always works out to thirty-seven (see the translator's introduction, Cheng, 1965/1999: x).

12 See Davis & Mann's (1996) informative interview with Benjamin Lo, Professor Zheng's first student in Taiwan and standard-bearer in the United States.

13 The name Shizhong (Shih Chung, as it was first romanized in Taibei, or Shr Jung as it was later transliterated by the American branch in New York City) refers to the ideas of correct timing and balance and resonates with literary allusions to the *Doctrine of the Mean* and other classics of traditional Chinese literature and philosophy, with which Zheng was well versed.

14 See Robert W. Smith's classic text (1974/1990), and the follow-up memoir (1999), for details on that pioneering martial historian's adventures in Taiwan. See also Mason (2001) for an extensive interview with Smith.

15 For details see translator Tam Gibbs's "Brief Biography of Professor M. C. Cheng" in the Professor's commentary on Laozi (Cheng, 1971/1981: 239).

16 According to an internet announcement circulated by Bill Law of the Melbourne Cheng Zi Taichi Chuan Study Association (2/15/02), Ju Hongbin, who teaches extensively in southern Taiwan as well as at the Taibei Shizhong, dedicated a separate memorial hall to the memory of Zheng in Gaoxiong on September 23, 2001. The flat is located at 2/F, 255 Ming Hua Rd., in the Gu Shan District of Gaoxiong.

17 In 1982 the National Palace Museum, in cooperation with Madame Zheng, put on a special retrospective exhibit of more than two dozen of Professor Zheng's paintings and calligraphic works. This was an outstanding honor, as the museum rarely featured the work of modern artists. A catalogue of prints was published

along with a preface previously written by Madame Chiang Kai-shek, who had been a painting student of Professor Zheng (Davis, 1996: 48).

[18] For more information see "Interview with Grand Master Hsu Yee Chung," edited by Massimiliano Biondi and published on the Shizhong Study Society webpage at: www.37taichi.org.tw

[19] More details of the opening ceremony may be found in the *Zheng Manqing Memorial Hall Donors' Record* booklet, published by the association in 2007.

Acknowledgements

Thanks are in order to all those who contributed to this project in ways large and small. Xu Yizhong gave his enthusiastic support and gracious permission to use photographs and materials. Benjamin Lo, Robert W. Smith, Liu Xiheng, Yuan Weiming, and Danny Emerick provided photos and other assistance, as did Monica Chen, Julia Fairchild, Ken Van Sickle, Mark Westcott, and others. A special debt of gratitude is owed Nick Tan and Jeff Herrod (as well as other researchers noted in the bibliography) for help with the translation of source materials. Readers' corrections are welcome. The author would like to acknowledge the late Tam Gibbs and to thank Ed Young and Maggie Newman for their help and encouragement. For more information on the Master Zheng Taijiquan Study Association, please contact via their website: www.37taichi@yahoo.com.tw.

Bibliography

Barnstone T., & Chou, P. (1996). *The art of writing: Teachings of the Chinese masters*. Boston: Shambhala.

Biondi, M. (2006). Interview with grand master Hsu Yee Chung. Published on the Shizhong Study Society webpage at www.37taichi.org.tw

Chen, W. (1929/1985). *T'ai chi ch'uan ta wen: Questions and answers on t'ai chi ch'uan* (B. Lo, & R. Smith, Trans.). Berkeley, CA: North Atlantic Books.

Cheng, M. (1962). *T'ai chi ch'uan: A simplified method of calisthenics for health and self defense*. Taibei: Shizhong Taijiquan Center.

Cheng, M. (1965/1999). *Master Cheng's new method of taichi ch'uan self-cultivation* (M. Hennessy, Trans.). Berkeley, CA: Frog, Ltd.

Cheng, M., & Smith, R. (1967/2004). *T'ai chi*. Rutland, VT: Charles E. Tuttle.

Cheng, M. (1971/1981). *Lao-tzu: My words are very easy to understand* (T. Gibbs, Trans.). Berkeley, CA: North Atlantic Books.

Cheng, M. (1985). *Cheng Tzu's thirteen treatises on t'ai chi ch'uan* (B. Lo & M. Inn, Trans.). Richmond, CA: North Atlantic Books.

Cheng, M. (1996). *T'ai chi ch'uan: A simplified method of calisthenics for health and self defense*. [Video]. Ashville, NC: Cho San.

Chengtzu Tai-Chi Chuan Research Association, (2007). *Cheng Man-ch'ing Ji Nien Guan donors' record*. Taibei, Taiwan.

Davis, B. (1996). In search of a unified Dao: Zheng Manqing's life and contributions to taijiquan. *Journal of Asian martial arts*, 5(2), 36–59.

Davis, D., & Mann, L. (1996). Conservator of the *Taiji classics*: An interview with Benjamin Pang Jeng Lo. *Journal of Asian martial arts*, 5(4), 46–67.

Fairchild, J., & Lin, G. (2007). The beginnings, growth, and development of taijiquan in Taiwan: An interview with Chairman Wang Yennien. Taibei, Taiwan: Yen-nien Shanghao, published on the Yen-nien Daoguan website.

Hayward, R. (1993). *T'ai-chi ch'uan: Lessons with master T. T. Liang*. St. Paul, MN: Shukuang Press.

Jou, T. (1981/1991). *The Tao of tai-chi chuan: Way to rejuvenation*. Warwick, NY: Tai Chi Foundation.

Lo, B., Inn, M., Amacker, R., & Foe, S. (1979). *The essence of t'ai chi ch'uan: The literary tradition*. Richmond, CA: North Atlantic Books.

Mason, R. (2001). Fifty years in the fighting arts: An interview with Robert W. Smith. *Journal of Asian martial arts*, 10(1), 36–73.

Mason, R. (2006). Review of the book *Yang Chengfu: The essence and applications of taijiquan*. *Journal of Asian martial arts*, 15(3), 92–93.

Smith, R. (1974/1990). *Chinese boxing: Masters and methods*. Berkeley, CA: North Atlantic Books.

Smith, R. (1975). A master passes: A tribute to Cheng Man-ch'ing. *Shr Jung newsletter*, 1(1), 2–7.

Smith, R. (1995). Remembering Zheng Manqing: Some sketches from his life. *Journal of Asian martial arts*, 4(3), 46–59.

Smith, R. (1999). *Martial musings: A portrayal of martial arts in the 20th century*. Erie, PA: Via Media.

Wile, D. (1985). *Cheng Man-Ch'ing's advanced t'ai-chi form instructions*. Brooklyn, NY: Sweet Ch'i Press.

Wile, D. (2007). *Zheng Manqing's uncollected writings on taijiquan, qigong, and health, with new biographical notes*. Milwaukee, WI: Sweet Ch'i Press.

Yang, C. (1934/2005). *Yang Chengfu: The essence and applications of taijiquan* (L. Swaim, Trans.). Berkeley, CA: North Atlantic Books.

Yang, J. (2001). *Tai chi secrets of the Yang style*. Boston, MA: YMAA Publication Center.

Yang, Z. (1988). *Yang style taijiquan*. Hong Kong: Hai Feng Publishing Co. and Beijing, China: Morning Glory Press.

Yang, Z. (1993). *Yang Cheng Fu shi tai ji quan*. Guangxi Province, China: Guangxi Minzu.

Yu, W., & Sharp, G. (1993). Fu Zhongwen: A Yang family legend. *Inside kung-fu*, April 1993, 44–46.

index

Analects 12, 18, 20, 125, 178
Art of Taijiquan, 88, 93
Art of War; Sunzi 18, 160
Attaining Softness Taijiquan Society (*zhi rou*) 5, 88
automatic writing 81, 82
Beijing 4, 5, 15, 56, 77, 78, 87, 88, 90, 91, 172, 173, 181
Book of Changes (*Yijing, I Ching*) 5, 12, 13, 18
Buddhism 76, 114, 122, 125, 130, 132–135, 138
Cai, Yuanpei 5, 172
Central Military Academy (Huangpu, Whampoa) 6, 124, 176
Cernuschi Museum of Chinese Art 9, 62, 178
Chen, "Tacky" Hanqiang 72, 73
Chen, Panling 177
Chen taijiquan 15, 150, 151, 165
Chen, Weiming 5, 6, 15, 17, 53, 55, 56, 58, 59, 60, 80, 86–100, 149, 153, 164, 165, 174, 175
Chen, Xing 149
Chen, Zhangxing 89, 149, 151
Chen, Zichen (William C. C. Chen) 35, 36, 40, 54, 180
Chenjiagou (Chen Village) 57, 88, 89, 90
Chiang, Kai-shek 6, 11, 13, 174, 176, 178
Chiang, Kai-shek, Madam 7, 14, 34
Chongqing 6, 69, 70, 72, 74, 75, 79, 95
College of Chinese Culture 7
Confucius 2, 4, 10, 11, 13, 18, 57, 63, 82, 107, 125, 132, 152, 161, 171
dalü (see large rollback)
Dao 1, 2, 5, 10, 13, 18, 50, 74, 113, 114, 115, 133, 137
Daoism, Daoist 53, 55, 60, 74, 75, 108, 130, 148, 152, 159, 160, 164
Daodejing 5, 10, 11, 18, 33, 159, 178
dianxue (art of attacking vital points) 74, 80
Ding, Yidu 6, 173
dispersing hands (*sanshou*) 39, 45, 46, 101
Dong, Yingjie 15, 54, 56, 77, 96
Emerick, Danny 69, 85, 139–144
energy work (*qi, qigong*) 13, 34, 41, 45, 46, 51, 60, 69, 72, 76, 79, 89, 93, 131, 133, 156, 160, 161
Essence and Applications of Taijiquan 113, 174, 175
FAR Gallery 62, 178
force (*li*) 55, 56, 60, 69, 77, 88, 89, 93, 97, 115, 131, 133, 137, 143, 160
Fu, Zhongwen 176
Gibbs, Tam 13, 59, 60, 69, 81, 109, 186
Guo, Qinfang 69, 70, 71, 73, 76, 77, 82, 85
Hall of Happiness 186
Han, Qingtang 177

Hangzhou 4, 172
health 1, 10, 14, 15, 16, 17, 18, 37, 61, 78, 117, 118, 119, 120, 136, 148, 153, 173, 186
Hong, Shihao 77
Huang, Xingxian 38–40, 47, 52, 54, 60
Hudson River Museum 10, 62, 178
Hunan Martial Arts Academy 6, 50, 75, 124, 153, 176
internal strength (*jin*) 32, 160, 161
Japan 4–6, 136, 141, 172, 176
Ju, Hongbin 124, 136, 180
Ke, Qihua 124, 132, 180
Koh, Ahtee 42, 43
large rollback (*dalü*) 93, 101–112
li (see force)
Li, Shoujian 102, 110, 111
Li, Xiheng 52, 69, 85, 113–147, 176–178, 182, 189, 193
Li, Yaxuan 174
Liang, Tongcai 32, 102, 103, 105–108, 136
Lin, Sen 173
Lo, Benjamin Pangjeng 52–54, 59, 85, 95, 97, 99, 102–107, 118–122, 128, 148–169
Lowenthal, Wolfe 60, 132, 158
Lu, Tongbao 38, 39, 41, 42, 44, 47, 54, 60
Luo, Banzhen (see Lo, Benjamin)
Malaysia 31–48, 49, 52, 60
Manran San Lun 12, 32, 96
Mao, Zedong 10, 11
Master Cheng's New Method of T'ai Chi Ch'uan Self-Cultivation 8
Master of Five Excellences 3, 152, 170, 171, 173
Master Zheng Taijiquan Study Association 117, 124, 180, 182, 193
Nanjing 6, 51, 83
National Association for Practitioners of Traditional Chinese Medicine 153, 173
National Chinese Medical Association 6, 118, 171, 173
National Palace Museum 14, 181
National Zhinan University 5
neigong (internal work) 34, 51, 132, 148
New York 1, 9–11, 13, 14, 58–62, 69, 81, 114, 121, 130, 154, 178, 180
Ng, Kionghing 37
Paris 9, 10, 62, 178
push-hands (*tuishou*) 33, 34, 40, 41, 44–46, 51–54, 56, 59–63, 76, 78, 80, 86, 93, 96, 101–103, 113, 114, 117, 119, 127–129, 131, 133, 137, 138, 143, 157–160, 176, 178, 179, 182
qi, qigong (see energy work)
Qian, Mingshan 5, 96

195

Questions and Answers on Taiji Boxing 55, 149
Republic of China Cultural Renaissance 11, 178
sanshou (see dispersing hands)
ROC Chinese Boxing Association 177
Shanghai 5, 52, 70, 73, 76–78, 86, 88, 96, 172, 173
Shanghai School of Fine Arts 5, 172
Shi, Shufang 72
Shizhong (Shr Jung, Shih Chung) 8–10, 13, 114, 117, 121, 124, 126, 130, 131, 136, 137, 139, 177, 178, 180, 181, 185, 189
Shaolin 33, 38
Singapore 14, 38, 39, 43, 44, 54, 180
Sino-Japanese War 6, 14, 16, 59, 60, 70, 95, 96, 135, 136, 153, 173, 175, 176
Smith, Robert W. 8, 19, 36, 132, 142, 152, 155, 159
Song, You'an 5, 173
Song, Zijian 33, 34, 39
sticking energy (*zhan*) 34, 92, 102, 157
Sun Lutang 57, 87, 88
Sutton, Nigel 49, 50, 54, 55, 58–64, 152, 161
T'ai Chi 8
Taiji: A Scientific Approach 136, 144, 149, 151, 156, 157
Taiji Classics 55, 61, 63, 78, 95, 102, 115, 133, 144, 149, 151, 156, 157
Taijiquan for Health and Self-Defense 8
Taiji Sword 88, 89
Taijiquan Academic Research Committee 177
taiji sword / taiji jian 13, 34, 45, 46, 88, 89, 113, 130, 154, 155, 183
Tan, Chingngee 43, 45
Tay, Guanleong 45, 46
tuberculosis 5, 33, 86, 152, 173, 174
tuishou (see push-hands)
United Nations 7, 9
Wan, Laisheng 50, 51, 75
Wang, Langting 92
Wang, Yangming 18, 50
Wang, Xiuai 69
Wang, Yannian 50–52, 78, 114, 182
Wang, Zongyue 57, 151
Waterside Pavilion, Beijing 172
Wenzhou 3, 38, 171
women 9, 14, 17
Wu, Guozhong 35, 38, 39, 41–44, 47, 53, 54, 58
Wu, Jianquan 53, 57
Wu, Mengxia 75
Wu, Tunan 56, 150
Xu, Yizhong 69, 75, 76, 85, 114, 121, 123–127, 132, 136–138, 146, 176, 180–182, 189, 193
Wudang Mountain 89, 148, 164
Xu, Zhengmei 134–139, 146
Xiong, Yangho 177

Xu, Chongming 182
Yang, Banhou 54, 56, 57, 89–92, 149
Yang, Chengfu 5, 6, 15, 17, 31–33, 50, 52–58, 60, 77, 78, 80, 86–89, 93, 111, 113, 124, 149, 152, 153, 160, 174–176
Yang, Jianhou 50, 56, 57, 89, 92, 149
Yang, Luchan 15, 51, 56, 57, 88–92, 149, 151, 152, 159, 162
Yang, Shaohou 56, 57, 88, 89
Yijing (*I Ching*, see *Book of Changes*) 5, 12, 13, 18, 33, 159, 160, 178
Yuan, Weiming 126–134, 146, 189, 193
Yue, Shuting 38–41, 44, 60
Yuwen University 5, 172
Zhan, Deshen 181
Zhang, Qinlin 51, 52, 59, 78
Zhang, Qingling 33
Zhang, Guan 3
Zhang, Sanfeng 43, 89, 148, 150, 151, 187
Zheng, Manqing
  birth 3, 171, 181, 187
  calligraphy 3, 4, 7, 12–14, 32, 37, 56, 108, 121, 125, 152, 153, 170–172, 181, 183–185
  death 2, 3, 13, 14, 35, 36, 81, 130, 180
  father 3
  grandmother 4
  illness 3, 4, 152, 172, 174
  intelligence 3, 172, 173
  mother 3, 5, 8, 172, 173
  painting 3–5, 7–14, 32, 73, 108, 118, 149, 152, 153, 170–173, 178, 181, 185, 187, 188
  poetry 2–5, 7, 8, 12, 19, 149, 152, 153, 170–172
  publications 3, 5, 6, 8, 9, 12, 13, 17, 32, 36, 53, 63, 102, 121, 122, 125, 174, 175, 181
  taijiquan teaching methods 1, 10, 16, 18, 31, 34–36, 55, 62, 63, 154
  thirty-seven-posture form 6, 17, 32–34, 54, 57, 101, 113, 124, 139, 142, 149, 176, 178
  traditional culture 2, 6, 9–11, 113
  wife (Juliana T. Zheng, Ding Yidu) 6, 69, 173
Zheng Manqing Memorial Hall 124, 170, 181, 182, 188
Zheng, Patrick 80, 81, 85, 155
Zhongshan Hall 118, 119, 125, 136, 176
Zuo Laipeng 32, 34, 40, 50–53, 59, 161

www.ingramcontent.com/pod-product-compliance
Lightning Source LLC
Chambersburg PA
CBHW071437080526
44587CB00014B/1882